NUTRITION AND DIET RESEARCH PROGRESS

VITAMIN D DEFICIENCY

Nutrition and Diet Research Progress

Additional books in this series can be found on Nova's website
under the Series tab.

Additional E-books in this series can be found on Nova's website
under the E-book tab.

NUTRITION AND DIET RESEARCH PROGRESS

VITAMIN D DEFICIENCY

VLADIMIR LERNER
AND
CHANOCH MIODOWNIK
EDITORS

Nova Science Publishers, Inc.
New York

For permission to use material from this book please contact us:
Telephone 631-231-7269; Fax 631-231-8175
Web Site: http://www.novapublishers.com

Additional color graphics may be available in the e-book version of this book.

Library of Congress Cataloging-in-Publication Data

Vitamin D deficiency / editors, Vladimir Lerner and Chanoch Miodownik.
p. ; cm.
Includes bibliographical references and index.
ISBN 978-1-61470-964-0 (hardcover)
I. Lerner, Vladimir. II. Miodownik, Chanoch.
[DNLM: 1. Vitamin D Deficiency--complications. WD 145]
LC classification not assigned
615.3'28--dc23

2011028968

Published by Nova Science Publishers, Inc. † New York

Contents

Preface

Since 1922 till now, according to PubMed, more than 50,000 articles regarding vitamin D were published. During last years the amount of publications about this topic significantly increases. Only through 2010 about 3000 articles were published.

Vitamin D is a secosteroid (its active form 1,25-$(OH)_2$-Vitamin D_3) a fat-soluble vitamin and a hormone precursor that plays an important role in bone metabolism and seems to have some anti-inflammatory and immune-modulating properties. It appears to have an effect on numerous diseases and disorders, including osteoporosis, chronic musculoskeletal pain, diabetes (types 1 and 2), multiple sclerosis, cardiovascular disease, and cancers of the breast, prostate, and colon. Although it is well known fact that combination of vitamin D and calcium is necessary to maintain bone density as people age, vitamin D may also be an independent risk factor for falls among the elderly. Most cells and tissues in the human body have vitamin D receptors that stimulate the nuclear transcription of various genes to alter cellular function. Since vitamin D not only affects the expression of many genes, but also has intra-individual pharmacokinetic variation, a simplistic cause and effect between vitamin D deficiency and illnesses should not be expected. During last decades, a dramatic increase occurred in our understanding of many biological actions result from vitamin D acting. New data were accumulated regarding a worldwide vitamin D deficiency in various populations, including infants, elderly, pregnant and lactating women.

The purpose of this book is to introduce the importance of vitamin D and its deficiency in all over human being life. Although, vitamin D is known to be a cardinal issue for years, in the last decade many new data were accumulated. The book contains 9 chapters and a commentary in which the authors try to summarize some of the most interesting and important subjects where vitamin D plays a role.

Chapter I presents an update review regarding low levels of vitamin D, which were evaluated by assessing 25OHD levels and authors individual clinical and experimental investigations on vitamin D insufficiency/deficiency. There is a general agreement regarding the increase in vitamin D deficiency, which can be evaluated by assessing 25OHD levels. Attaining adequate vitamin D nutritional status is important not only from a nutritional point of view, but also to ensure the effectiveness of anticatabolic treatments. The levels of 25OHD and parathyroid hormone (PTH) follow an inverse correlation and the point at which it reaches a plateau has been used to identify the lowest 25OHD threshold level. However, the critical reference range of 25OHD levels to ensure the endocrine and paracrine functions of vitamin D for overall health and well being is controversial. In addition, it is necessary to know at which point calcium intake could alter this range. Nevertheless, an important matter that must be taken into account is the difficulties related to 25OHD assay. Indeed, interlaboratories results differ greatly. One of the reasons might be the fact that circulating levels of 25OHD are the sum of two compounds of different origin: D_3 or cholecalciferol and D_2 or ergocalciferol. In this regard, there are several methods to measure 25OHD levels that vary in accuracy and sensitivity and not all detect the two compounds simultaneously.

Chapter II is an overview of available data on extra-skeletal effects of vitamin D deficiency and available interventional studies. Available data support the notion that vitamin D deficiency is both an independent risk factor, at least for some extra-skeletal diseases, and a non-specific marker of poor health.

Chapter III deals with vitamin D and its connection to hypertension. Adequate vitamin D levels are necessary for good vascular health. Vitamin D, in addition to increasing intestinal calcium absorption, reducing parathyroid hormone levels and improving the amount and quality of bone, has a beneficial vascular effect. Vitamin D deficiency has been associated with arterial hypertension. This association between hypertension and vitamin D deficit is mediated by activation of the renin-angiotensin-aldosterone system. High calcitriol levels reduce plasma renin activity, leading to reduced plasma angiotensin II concentrations. This modulation of the renin-angiotensin-aldosterone system, besides reducing blood pressure, decreases inflammation in the vascular endothelium, limiting the progression of atherosclerosis.

In Chapter IV present accumulated data regarding vitamin D deficiency and its relationship on cardiovascular disease. Vitamin D has pluripotent cardiovascular effects, where the activity of its receptors have been affiliated to blood pressure regulation through inhibition of vascular smooth muscle proliferation, down regulation of myocyte proliferation and their hypertrophy, cardiac muscle contractility, decrease in plasma renin activity, anti-inflammatory properties, as well cholesterol synthesis and hydroxylation. Vitamin D supplementation in the intent to lower cardiovascular outcomes however, has not been convincingly shown as beneficial. Thus despite the promise for disease prevention suggested by available studies, the evidence for widespread use of high-dose vitamin D supplementation in the general population remains insufficient. The cardiovascular risk associated with vitamin D deficiency has been demonstrated regardless of the amount of solar exposure suggesting the possibility that vitamin D deficiency could be a biomarker of a passive life style rather than the cause of increased CVD risk.

The prevalence of hypovitaminosis D is high in patients with osteoporotic hip fracture. Chapter V summarizes the role of vitamin D deficiency in patients with osteoporotic hip fracture. Hip fracture is associated with a high morbidity and mortality, and represents a major health problem in developed countries. Vitamin D deficiency has a high prevalence among these patients, and it seems to be associated with several factors, related to the patient and/or the type of the fracture. Some studies have suggested that patients with throchanteric fractures are older, have a poor pre-fracture health status and a higher prevalence of hypovitaminosis D. The osteoporotic hip fracture has a seasonal presentation, with a lower incidence in summer, that correlates with higher levels of $25(OH)D_3$ and a higher solar radiation in the previous months.

Vitamin D is not just for preventing rickets and osteomalacia. Recent findings in animal experiments, epidemiologic studies and clinical trials indicate that adequate vitamin D levels are important for cancer prevention. Chapter VI highlights the role of vitamin D in nutritional imprinting and reviews the current literature on vitamin D deficiency and the pathogenesis of breast and prostate cancer. The fetal-origin hypothesis has reshaped the way of scientific thinking by identifying that the prenatal metabolic environment can be memorized by the developing organism through fetal and neonatal imprinting. In light of this hypothesis, prenatal events can be thought of as the foundation for structural and functional development of an organism. Altered endocrine expression and/or nutritional inadequacy during development are two forms of metabolic disruptions that may have long-term consequences for health. Specifically, vitamin D inadequacy during pregnancy and early postnatal life has been associated with an increased risk for nutritional rickets, failure to thrive, osteomalacia and osteoporosis. Emerging evidence also suggests that long-term vitamin D inadequacy is implicated in many chronic diseases including cancer.

The high prevalence of vitamin D deficiency during childhood is of major public health concern. Vitamin D deficiency is quite common among children and adolescents in the United States and worldwide. Chapter VII is focused on definitions, epidemiology, clinical implications, and treatment of vitamin D deficiency in children and adolescents. Early identification, treatment, and prevention of vitamin D deficiency in childhood may have profound health effects throughout life span.

Chapter VIII discusses the prevalence of vitamin D insufficiency in the elderly, describe the negative effects of a lack of this vitamin on the health of older people, and relate to the possible beneficial effects of vitamin D supplementation in the older population. Prevalence studies have demonstrated that its deficiency is widespread among the older population worldwide. While the effects of inadequate levels of vitamin D on calcium metabolism and the development of osteoporosis are well known among health care providers, there is mounting evidence for other consequences of a lack of this vitamin on the health of the elderly. Studies have shown that insufficient levels of vitamin D are associated with functional disability and falls at an advanced age.

The central nervous system is increasingly being recognized as a target organ for vitamin D via its wide-range steroid hormonal effects and via the induction of various proteins such as nerve growth factor. Vitamin D is notably associated with the pathology of cognition and mental illnesses. Vitamin D receptors have been detected on neurons that regulate behaviour. Chapter IX deals with vitamin D serum concentration in patients with major depression and schizophrenia in comparison to healthy controls in order to determine if a correlation exists between serum levels of vitamin D and mental conditions. Lower serum vitamin D levels were found in patients with schizophrenia compared to patients with depression or healthy controls.

In this book is presented a commentary regarding vitamin D levels in patients with Paget's disease of bone (PDB). Hypocalcemia and secondary hyperparathyroidism have been described after treatment with bisphosphonates in various conditions, including osteoporosis, bone metastases and PDB. Hypocalcemia seems to be more severe after treatment with the more potent, intravenous bisphosphonates, including zoledronic acid, which is currently the treatment of choice for PDB.

Though much has been written about vitamin D deficiency, this clearly is not a new problem. Awareness of the medical morbidities as a result of vitamin D deficiency is a vital step towards intervention in the pathological process. Furthermore, this will help to protect and prevent serious complications and finally greater access to clinicians in all areas of medicine.

We believe that a better understanding of vitamin D deficiency will strengthen the efforts and success of diagnose and treat this condition effectively.

In: Vitamin D Deficiency
Editors: V. Lerner and C. Miodownik

ISBN: 978-1-61470-964-0

Chapter I

Update on Low Levels of 25OHD and Outcomes: Our Experience

***Susana Noemi Zeni**[*1,2]*
***and Maria Luz Pita Martin de Portela**[3]*
[1] Osteopaties Medical Section of Clinical Hospital "J. de San Martín". School of Medicine. Buenos Aires University, Argentina
[2] National Council of Technical and Scientific Research. Argentina (CONICET), Argentina
[3] Nutrition Department. School of Pharmacy and Biochemistry. Buenos Aires University, Argentina

Abstract

There is a general agreement regarding the increase on vitamin D deficiency which can be evaluated by assessing the levels of 25OHD. To achieve an adequate vitamin D nutritional status is important not only by a nutritional point of view, but also for the effectiveness of anticatabolic treatments. The levels of 25OHD and PTH follow an inverse correlation where the point at which it reaches a plateau has been used to identify a lower 25OHD threshold level. However, the critical reference range of 25OHD levels to ensure the endocrine and paracrine functions of vitamin D for overall health and well being is controversial. In addition, it is necessary to know at which point calcium intake could alter this range. However, an important question to be taken into account is the difficulties related to the 25OHD assay. Indeed, the results informed by several laboratories are very different for a same concentration of 25OHD. One of the reasons can be explained by the fact that circulating levels of 25OHD are the sum of two compounds of different origin: D_3 or cholecalciferol and D_2 or ergocalciferol. In this regard, there are several methods to measure 25OHD levels that varying in accuracy and sensitivity and not all of them detect simultaneously the two compounds. The objective of

[*] Correspondence: Prof. Dr. Susana Zeni, Córdoba 2351 – 8vo. Piso Ciudad de Buenos Aires, Argentina, TEL-FAX.: 541159508972 Email: snzeni@hotmail.com.

the present review is to make an update on these issues and to share our clinical and experimental investigations on vitamin D insufficiency/deficiency.

Keywords: Inadequacy – vitamin D – 25hydroxyvitamin D – hypovitaminosis D

Abbreviations

AAOMM	Argentine Association of Osteology and Mineral Metabolism
AI	Adequate Intake
BA -	Buenos Aires
BMD	bone mineral density
Ca	calcium
CLIA	chemiluminescence
CV	coefficient of variation
DBP	Vitamin D Binding Protein
DEQAS	External Quality Assessment Scheme
DRI	Dietary Reference Intakes
EARs	Estimated Average Requirements
EIA	enzymatic immunoassays
FGF23	fibroblast growth factor 23
GCMS	gas chromatography mass spectrometry
HPLC	high performance liquid chromatography
2°HPT	secondary hyperparathyroidism
IMNAS-	Institute of Medicine of the National Academy of Sciences
IGF1	Insulin Growth Factor 1
IU	International Units
LC–MS/MS	Liquid Chromatography Tandem Mass Spectroscopy
M	Postmenopausal women
ng/ml	nanograms/mililiter
nmol/L	nanomole/liter
NIST	National Institute of Standards and Technology
$1,25(OH)_2D$	calcitriol
25OHD	25-hydroxyvitamin D
P	Phosphorus
pg/ml	picograms/mililiter
PM	Premenopausal women
PTH	Parathormone
RDAs	Recommended Dietary Allowances
RIA	radioimmunoassay
S	South latitude
SD	standard deviation
SHAM	simulated surgery
UVB	Ultraviolet B light
ys	years

Introduction

Metabolism of Vitamin D

Vitamin D, from a nutritional point of view, is an atypical nutrient because, when the exposure to sunlight is adequate, most of the total vitamin D requirement of white people can be obtained by the skin photoconversion. Indeed, skin exposure to ultraviolet B (UVB) light (280-315nm wavelength) synthesizes, in several non-enzymatic steps, vitamin D_3 or cholecalciferol from 7-dehydrocholesterol. Vitamin D can also be provided by dietary sources such as dairy products, eggs and fish as vitamin D_3, or from yeast and plants consumption as vitamin D_2 or ergocalciferol [1]. Both forms have been commercially synthesized and have been used to fortify foods or as supplements. Whatever the source of vitamin D, it must be metabolized twice before regulating calcium (Ca) and phosphorus (P) homeostasis. Native vitamin D is considered a preprohormone which is transported to the liver where a hepatic 25-hydroxilase transforms vitamin D into 25-hydroxyvitamin D (25OHD) or calcidiol. It is important to take into account that this hepatic enzyme metabolizes both, vitamin D_2 and D_3, equally efficiently into $25OHD_2$ and $25OHD_3$, respectively [2]. Then, total concentration of 25OHD in circulation is the sum of these two metabolites [3-4]. In the kidney proximal tubule 25OHD is converted by the renal 1α,25-hydroxilase into $1,25(OH)_2D$ or calcitriol, the active form of vitamin D [5].

Calcitriol functions as a hormone circulating in the blood to stimulate the net Ca absorption by the induction of various components of the Ca transport system in the intestinal mucosa. Severe vitamin D deficiency causes impairment of skeletal mineralization resulting in rickets in children and osteomalacia in adults [6]. Less severe degrees of vitamin D insufficiency contribute to reduce Ca absorption causing a secondary hyperparathyroidism (2°HPT) which increases bone turnover leading, over time, to bone loss without necessarily impairing bone mineralization [7,8].

Besides the kidney, many other tissues including osteoclast, skin, macrophages, placenta, colon, brain, prostate, endothelium and parathyroid glands express 1α,25-hydroxilase which can synthesize $1,25(OH)_2D$ locally [9]. This extrarenal production of calcitriol acts in an autocrine-paracrine way regulating up to 200 genes, which helps to control cell growth, cellular differentiation and immune function and may be responsible for decreasing the risk of the cells of being transformed into a malignant state [10]. In this regard, adequate vitamin D nutritional status is also recognized as convenient for vitamin D biological function in preventing a wide variety of conditions besides its role in bone fractures [11], among them: resistance to microbial infections [12], cardiovascular disease [13,14], diabetes [15], cancer [16] and asthma [17,18].

Biochemical Index of Nutritional Vitamin D Status

As the number of adverse health consequences associated with a low or even high vitamin D status increase it becomes imperative to determine vitamin D adequacy. Routine measurement of serum Ca and P provides no information about vitamin D status. The assessment of its physiological status by the amount of vitamin D provided by the sun and/or food is difficult. Measurements of sun exposure duration and intensity are complicated because they vary with age, latitude, season, time of the day, skin pigmentation, cloud cover or fraction of the body exposure, sunscreens use, body mass index and the amount of body fat [19]. In addition, although humans are physiologically capable of covering vitamin D adequacy through sunlight exposure, there are public health recommendations regarding the need to limit sun exposure to avoid cancer risk.

There are three main vitamin D metabolites circulating in the bloodstream bound to the vitamin D binding protein (DBP): native vitamin D, 25OHD and $1,25(OH)_2D$ and one of them is the optimal biochemical index of vitamin D nutritional status. Native vitamin D appears in the plasma for only a short period of time because of its rapid metabolism in the liver or storage in adipose tissue. The levels of $1,25(OH)_2D$ have little value and can mislead the clinicians [20]. Indeed, as vitamin D deficiency increases the secretion of the parathyroid hormone (PTH) also increases. Because PTH is a potent positive regulator of the renal 1α,25hydroxilase, this 2°HPT results in an increment in circulating concentration of calcitriol. In addition, the renal enzyme is also highly regulated by other factors such as calcitriol, P, insulin growth factor 1 (IGF1), fibroblast growth factor 23 (FGF23) [21], estrogen; which maintain the circulating levels of calcitriol between a narrow and constant level. The extra-renal production of $1,25(OH)_2D$ is not regulated by PTH and, according to literature, there is no evidence that contributes to the normal circulating levels of calcitriol [22]. The hallmark for determining vitamin D status is the measurement of the circulating concentration of 25OHD because, conversely to the renal 1α,25 hydroxylase, the hepatic enzyme 25-hydroxilase is poorly regulated. This makes the levels of 25OHD increase with vitamin D cutaneous synthesis and intake, including supplements, and therefore providing an integrated assessment of vitamin D supply and body stores. This metabolite has a half-life shorter than vitamin D (24hr vs. 2-3 wk) but higher than $1,25(OH)_2D$ (24hr vs. 4hr). In addition, the concentration of 25OHD in circulation is similar to vitamin D and about 1000 times higher than $1,25(OH)_2D$ (ng/ml vs. pg/ml). The 25OHD metabolite has a much lower affinity for the vitamin D receptor than $1,25(OH)_2D$ but much higher affinity than vitamin D itself and, although calcitriol is the most effective vitamin D metabolite, an adequate serum 25OHD level is also necessary to achieve full physiological vitamin D activity. It is currently accepted that total 25OHD measurement is appropriate to judge vitamin D status; as such, separate quantification of $25OHD_2$ and $25OHD_3$ is not essential [23].

After recognizing that circulating 25OHD is the best indicator to differentiate vitamin D insufficiency, adequacy and toxicity [1, 19], it is necessary to define both, normal range and a safe levels of 25OHD. Indeed, safety is always an important consideration as well, when formulating recommendations for a nutrient intake. Excessive amounts of vitamin D are not available from UVB because its cutaneous production is limited; however, chronic toxicity may be possible for the indiscriminate consumption of supplements. As the metabolism of vitamin D into 25OHD is a largely unregulated metabolic step, an increment in vitamin D intake results in higher circulation 25OHD levels, although perhaps not in a linear manner [24]. Vitamin D intoxication results by high plasma levels of 25OHD rather than by a high plasma $1,25(OH)_2D$ [25]. Vitamin D toxicity caused hypercalcemia, vomiting, ectopic calcifications and lethality [4]. Reports of vitamin D toxicity are exceptional; there is no evidence of vitamin D intoxication in healthy adults up to 25OHD levels of 250nml//L or

100ng/ml (nmo/L = ng/ml x 2.5). In the present Chapter both, nmol/l or ng/ml will be indistinctly used (figure 1).

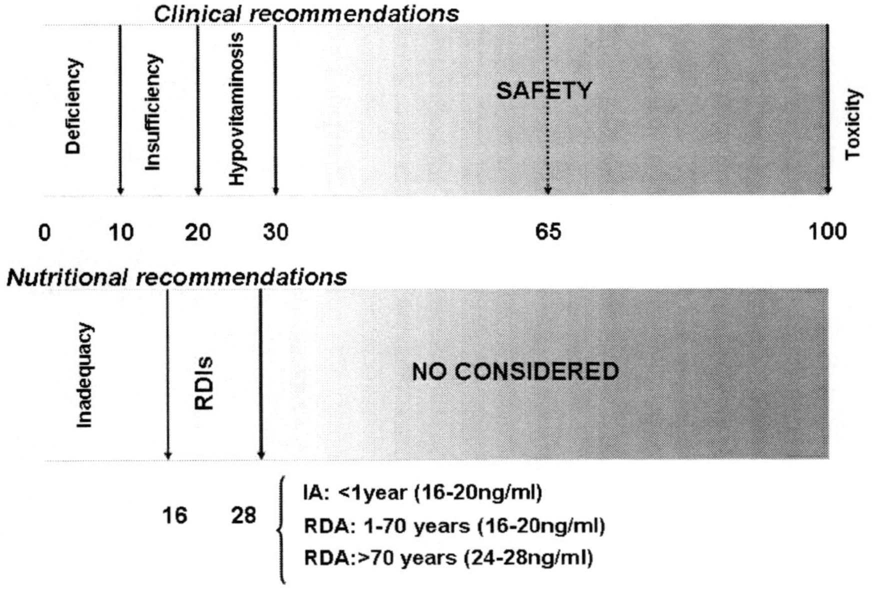

Figure 1. Comparative levels of 25OH (ng/ml) according to the clinical or nutritional recommendations.

The upper limit of 25OHD levels can be assume taking into account that healthy subject with a constantly high UVB exposure (e.g. lifeguards) reach levels of 25OHD (±2DS) of 163nmol/L or 65,2ng/ml [26]. On the other extreme, a deficiency of vitamin D is observed when circulating 25OHD levels are below 25nmol/L or 10ng/ml. This level puts the individual, depending on age, at risk of developing rickets and osteomalacia and delimits the lowest level to satisfy the body`s vitamin D requirement. Between upper and lower 25OHD values, some epidemiological and pharmacological studies suggest that there are two levels of vitamin D inadequacy. In this regard, hyperparathyroidism and high bone turnover are observed when 25OHD concentration is below 50 nmol/L or 20 ng/ml but higher than 25nmol/L or 10 mg/dl. These levels are considered insufficient because they may lead, over time, to osteoporosis and bone fractures [1] (figure 1). Such endocrine alterations were studied by Malabanan A et al [27] in 35 healthy adults who received 50.000IU of vitamin D during 8 weeks, with baseline circulating concentrations of 25OHD ranging between 10 and 25 ng/ml. They observed a 109% in increment in 25OHD levels while PTH decreased by approximately 40% when baseline concentrations of 25OHD ranged between 10 and 20ng/ml; however, no changes in PTH were observed when baseline 25OHD levels were higher than 20ng/ml. It is important to point out that inside this range of circulating 25OHD, the levels of calcitriol can be affected differently and they are often similar to or still higher than those of vitamin D-repleted subjects [28]. In this regard and according to clinical data, 25OHD levels of approximately 20nmol/L or 8ng/ml would be a critical value for the kidney production of calcitriol because of the synthesis of the active metabolite dependent on substrate availability, in the case of vitamin D deficiency [29].

Hypovitaminosis D can be defined as a condition where supplementation of exogenous vitamin D leads to a decrease of PTH concentrations. This level of inadequacy was suggested to be present when serum levels of 25OHD range between 50nmol/L and 75-80nmol/L or 20 and 30-32ng/ml; inside such range small increases in serum PTH could be observed, although within the normal limits [30, 31]; nevertheless, such increment might not be advantageous as it stimulates bone resorption. Indeed, when serum PTH concentration is plotted as a function of 25OHD levels an inverse function is observed in which PTH values rise as levels of 25OHD decrease. The curve flattens out above 25OHD values that range from 75 to 110nmol/L, depending on the report [4, 32-34]. A quasi-consensus of vitamin D and several researches proposed a threshold of circulating 25OHD concentrations of approximately 75nmol/L or 30ng/ml to avoid vitamin D-dependent body disturbances [35-37] (figure 1). This cut-off agrees with the value reported by Mc Kenna MJ and Freaney R [30] to define different states of vitamin D. In addition, according to several reports, this cut-off is also similar to that associated with: a) an increase in bone markers [38]; b) a maximal intestinal Ca absorption in postmenopausal women [39] or c) a diminution in fracture risk [40]. From epidemiological and interventional studies, several authors suggested a similar or close value [30-31, 41-42], but others proposed lower or higher cut-off than 30ng/ml. In this regard, Ooms et al [8] suggested that 2°HPT exists when 25OHD levels are lower than 30nmol/L or 12ng/ml [30, 43-44], while others reported that it is present at a threshold of 50nmol/L or 20ng/ml [45]; 62.5nmol/L or 25ng/ml [46]; or still higher: 110nmol/L or 44 ng/ml [47]. These differences could be partially explained by differences in ethnicity, Ca intake, age, latitude, clinical status or even the use of different assays to evaluate 25OHD levels. Recently, Heaney et al [48] suggested that the point at which hepatic 25OHD production becomes zero order could be used to define the lowest end of normal vitamin D status. Hepatic 25-hydroxylase appears to become saturated and the reaction switches from first to zero order when vitamin D exceeds approximately 5.8ng/ml. Taking this approach, the lowest normal limit is approximately 35ng/ml, quite close to the 30-32ng/ml suggested by other end points such as the relationship between 25OHD and PTH levels [49]. Moreover, it is worthy of emphasis that imprecision is present in all quantitative tests that evaluate 25OHD levels. Clearly, a value of 29ng/ml (72.5nmol/l) is not different from 30-32ng/ml (75-80nmol/l) and it should be considered to reflect optimal vitamin D status [23].

The 25OHD cutoff near 30ng/ml was obtained in researches conduced in postmenopausal women or in subjects older than 65 years (ys.) and, most of them, had studied the association between fracture incidence and vitamin D deficiency in which Ca supplementation was combined with vitamin D supplementation. Ca intake is an important point to consider because the threshold of 25OHD levels at which PTH levels begin to rise could be influenced by Ca intake. Low Ca intake induces an increase in serum PTH levels and decreases the half life of serum 25OHD both, in rats and in patients with partial gastrectomy, leading to vitamin D deficiency [50, 51]. In addition, Ca intake could influence the endpoints, such as hip fracture which is also affected by 25OHD concentrations [52].

Argentina is a large country that extends from latitude 22°S (La Puna) till 55°S (Ushuaia) while the capital city, Buenos Aires (BA), is located at 34°S allowing to divide the country into three regions: south, mid and north of similar ethnicity, diet and lifestyle. During 2003, the Research Committee of the Argentine Association of Osteology and Mineral Metabolism (AAOMM) conducted a large National research to study 'cutoff' 25OHD values above which serum PTH levels remained stable and relatively low [53]. The research included 386 ambulatory healthy Caucasian subjects over 65 ys. from 7 cities of Argentina between latitude 26ºS and 55ºS. The function between the levels of 25OHD and PTH showed a cut-off of 27ng/ml when all the studied population was included in the analysis (figure 2); moreover, if only the 169 subjects living in BA (34ºS) were included in the analysis the cut off was near 30ng/ml [54]. Both values are similar and agree with most clinical studies on bone health.

Dietary Recommended Intake of Vitamin D and Levels of 25OHD

The Committee of the Food and Nutrition Board of the Institute of Medicine, in 1997, considered circulating 25OHD as the functional indicator of vitamin D status; however, because of insufficient scientific data, the Committee members were unable to establish a specific level to estimate average requirements on which to set a dietary reference value for the Estimated Average Requirements (EARs) and for the Recommended Dietary Allowances (RDAs); these values, for definition, cover the needs for 50% and 97.5% of the population, respectively. So, they estimated a provisional recommendation for vitamin D intake and established an Adequate Intake (AI) of 5 μg/day for people between 1-50 ys., 10 μg/day for subjects' aged 50–70 years, and 15 μg/day for adults over 70 ys. of age [55].

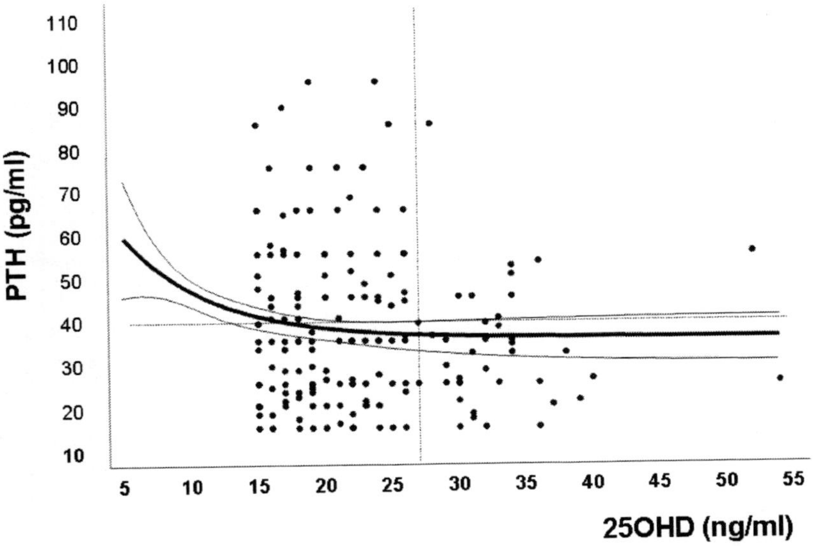

Figure 2. Individual levels of PTH (pg/ml) as a function of 25OHD (ng/ml) of 386 ambulatory healthy Caucasian subjects over 65 ys. from 7 cities of Argentina between latitude 26ºS and 55ºS. The threshold for 25OHD is 27ng/ml.

In 2010, the Institute of Medicine of the National Academy of Sciences (IMNAS) established the Dietary Reference Intakes (DRI) [56] for vitamin D based on the available evidence from data published between 1997 and 2009 [57, 58]. Although during such period, a great number of researches, which are increasing daily, suggest that vitamin D could potentially prevent or ameliorate acute and chronic non-skeletal diseases (e.g. diabetes, immune response, heart disease, cancer); the etiologies of these chronic diseases are generally multifactorial, where vitamin D would only be one of the involved factors. According to the

Committee, this makes difficult to choose one chronic disease as an endpoint to evaluate the effect of vitamin D. Then, because of the insufficient evidence to make any recommendations with respect to non-skeletal benefits, if any, the present DRI for vitamin D was only based on the effect on bone health and Ca absorption.

Although ignoring sunlight exposure may be inappropriate because for most people is a normal part of their lives, the concerns about skin cancer risk precluded incorporating the effect of sun exposure in the DRIs. On these bases, the Committee assumed that all vitamin D comes from the diet and recommended the measurement of serum 25OHD as a biomarker of exposure (i.e intake). In addition, they considered that the levels of this metabolite can reflect bone health outcomes under conditions of "minimal sun" exposure for USA and Canada population. The dose-response relationship between vitamin D intake and 25OHD levels were based on exploratory meta-regression analyses of the Agency of Health and Research of Quality, Ottawa (AHRQ-Ottawa). The AHRQ reported that there was a net change in serum 25OHD concentrations with increasing doses of vitamin D and found a rise between 1 and 2nmol/L or 0.4 to 0.8ng/mL in the levels for each additional 100 IU of vitamin D_3, both in children and in adults. However, the dose–response relationship differs depending on baseline serum 25OHD levels ($\leq$ 40 vs. > 40nmol/L) and supplementation duration ($\leq$ 3 vs. > 3 months) [59, 60].

The threshold of 25OHD near 30ng/ml for clinical interventions was not considered adequate for the members of the Committee to establish the dietary recommendations for vitamin D. Regarding this, they estimated that there is a considerable over-estimation of vitamin D deficiency percentage due to the use of some cut-points for serum 25OHD that greatly exceed the levels identified for the report. They concluded that a 25OHD concentration above 75nmol/L or 30ng/ml was not consistently associated with increase benefit and suggested that an ~20 ng/mL cut-off was enough to ensure bone health for most of the population indicating that it was uncertain about its extraskeletal benefits.

The standard model to establish DRIs was based on a normal distribution assumption for requirements and used the average or median to estimate EAR and added ±2SD to estimate RDA. A range of 25OHD between 40 to 50nmol/L or 16 to 20ng/mL was used to establish an AI of 400 IU (10µg) per day for infants. This range of 25OHD level was also used to specify an RDA of 600 IU (15µg) per day for children and adolescents (1 to 18 ys.) and for young adults and adults (19 through 50 ys.). The EAR and RDA for people older than 50 ys. and up to 70 ys. are the same as that for young adults. The analyses for establishing these recommendations were carried out according to the following evidences: a) there was a trend toward a maximal Ca absorption for both children and adults when 25OHD levels ranged between 30 and 50nmol/L or 12-20ng/m without clear evidence of further benefit above 50 nmol/L; b) when Ca intake was adequate, the risk of rickets increased below a serum 25OHD level of 30nmol/L and was minimal when serum 25OHD levels ranged between 30 and 50nmol/L; c) when Ca intake was inadequate, there was no effect of vitamin D supplementation to reach a serum 25OHD concentrations up to and beyond 75nmol/L or 30ng/mL; d) several researches suggested that serum 25OHD concentration of approximately 40nmol/L or 16ng/mL were enough to meet bone health requirements for most people; however, others found that levels of 50nmol/L or 20ng/ml and higher were consistent with bone health; e) Priemel et al. [61] in a *post-mortem observational study* regarding *osteomalacia* found that serum 25OHD level of 50nmol/L or 20ng/ml provided coverage for at least 97.5% of the population. Further, a higher level of 75nmol/L proposed as "optimal" and hence consistent with an RDA-type reference value was not well supported. For the elderly, serum 25OHD concentrations in the range of 60 to 70nmol/L or 24 to 28ng/ml were associated with the lowest risk of hip fracture suggesting that somewhat higher serum 25OHD concentrations were needed to provide maximum population coverage. Therefore, and taking into account factors such as changes in bone mineral density (BMD) and fracture risk, the RDA for people older than 70ys. was increased to 800 IU/day (20μg), level that exceeded the 2SD related to the other groups [56] (figure 1). The Committee accepted an "assay drift" associated with a longitudinal comparison of assay results of 25OHD levels collected by the analyses of the different reports for determining DRI; however, it also considered that this "assay drift" did not influence the established vitamin D recommendations.

Some researchers dissent with many of the findings and recommendations of this report [62, 63].

Inadequacy of Vitamin D

1. Prevalence

Although controversy remains over the optimal vitamin D cut-point to be used for a clinical diagnosis of vitamin D "inadequacy", there is increasing "clinical" consensus that values less than 30-32ng/ml are indicative of suboptimal vitamin D status [7, 37, 64]. In considering this value, vitamin D inadequacy measured by serum 25OHD levels is perhaps the most widespread deficiency condition in developed nations. It has been classified as an "epidemic"-affecting approximately 25%–35% of the US adult population [65] and up to 80% of high-risk populations such as dark-skinned individuals or those with limited/no sun exposure [66]. Other researchers also reported high levels of vitamin D inadequacy even in sunny countries [67-69]. In this regard, a recent published research reported high prevalence of vitamin D insufficiency (90%) in a group of 123 healthy adults (>20 years) living in Karachi, Pakistan [70].

The prevalence of 'vitamin D insufficiency' is well documented in traditional risk groups such as housebound, institutionalized, and elderly patients with hip fractures mainly due to a reduction in sun exposition or synthesis of vitamin D [71-73], but it is becoming increasingly recognized among the independent elderly, community-dwelling postmenopausal women and even in middle-aged subjects [7, 33, 37, 72, 74-76]. Insufficiency of vitamin D was also detected in other groups including newborns, infant and children, women during pregnancy and young adults [76, 77].

Several researches across different age groups were conducted in Argentina to evaluate vitamin D nutritional status.

a) Newborns and Their Mothers

The incidence of vitamin D inadequacy was evaluated in a 40 newborns and their mothers living in Ushuaia (n=16) and BA (n=24). The blood of the mothers was obtained after 24-48hr. postpartum and from the cord blood of their respective neonates. The mean levels of 25OHD were in Ushuaia: 6.3±4.8 and 3.9±2.7ng/ml in mothers and neonates, respectively, and in BA: 14.4±8.7 and 11.3±6.0ng/ml, respectively. Deficiency was observed in 75% of mothers and in 100% of neonates in Ushuaia and, in 38% and in 25% in BA, respectively. Insufficiency was observed in 25% of mothers and 0% of their neonates in Ushuaia while in BA the percentages were 46.5% and 62.5%, respectively. None of the mothers and their neonates reached levels of vitamin D adequacy in Ushuaia and only 2 mothers and 1 neonate in BA [78].

Vitamin D inadequacy according to the cut-off of 30ng/ml (clinical incidence) was observed in 100% of mothers and their neonates living in Ushuaia vs. 87.5% and 100%, respectively in those living in BA. When the cut-point for 25OHD was according to the DRI levels (RDI incidence) (<16ng/ml) inadequacy was: 81% and 100% in Ushuaia vs. 43% and 87.5% in BA, for mothers and neonates, respectively [78] (table 2).

b) Infants and Children

The National Survey of Nutrition and Health conducted by the Public Health Ministry of Argentina in 2004-2005 evaluated the 25OHD levels in 138 children aged 6 to 23 month from six provinces of the Patagonia at the beginning the summer. The mean 25OHD levels were 27.1±11.5ng/ml for the total region of Patagonia. Table 1 shows the mean value of 25OHD by province. No differences were found by socio-economic conditions [79]. Deficiency was 3.6%; insufficiency 27.5%; hypovitaminosis 42% and sufficiency 26.9%. The clinical incidence of vitamin D inadequacy was 73.1% while the DRI incidence was 16% (table 2).

Table 1. Sampling month, mean and confidence interval of the levels of 25OHD (ng/ml) obtained in138 children aged 6 to 23 month from six provinces of the Patagonia at the beginning of the summer

Province	Sampling Month	Mean (ng/mL)	CI to 95%	
Chubut (45°S)	October	26,6	24,9	28,2
Neuquén (38°S)	October	21,2	19,3	23,2
Santa Cruz (51°S)	November	27,0	24,2	29,8
Río Negro (40°S)	November	31,3	29,6	32,9
T. del Fuego (54°S)	December	32,1	29,8	34,3
La Pampa (36°S)	December	32,0	29,9	34,2

The vitamin D inadequacy was also investigated in healthy children from 4.0 to 9.0ys. living in three areas of Argentina: BA (n=37), Ushuaia (n=63) and Tucumán (26°S) (n=23). There were not differences in the mean value of 25OHD in BA and Tucuman (20.2±1.3 vs. 19.6±1.2ng/ml); however, the serum levels were significantly lower in Ushuaia as compared to the other two regions (9.3±0.6ng/ml). Deficiency was 14% in BA; 65% in Ushuaia and 0%

in Tucuman; insufficiency was 41%, 28% and 54.5% respectively; hipovitaminosis D was 28%, 7% and 41.5%, respectively and adequacy was17%, 0% and 0%, respectively [80].

The clinical incidence of vitamin D inadequacy was 83% in BA and 100% in both, Ushuaia and Tucumán. The DRI incidence of inadequacy was 38% in BA, 93% in Ushuaia and 23% in Tucumán (table 2).

Table 2. Summary of the studies mentioned in the text conducted in Argentina among people of different ages to determine the incidence of vitamin D inadequacy. Mean values of 25OHD are expressed in ng/ml; levels <10: deficiency; between 10 and <20: insufficiency; between 20 and <30 hypovitaminosis and >30 adequacy. Clinical: express the incidence of inadequacy taking a threshold of 30; DRI: express the incidence of inadequacy taking a threshold of 16 from newborn to adults of 70ys and 24 for adults >70 ys. Three different methodologies were employed. The references of the researches are given in the last column

	Mean value	Deficiency	Insuficiency	Hypovitam.	Adequacy	Clinical	DRI	Methodolgy	Ref.
Newborns BA	11-3±6.0	25	62,5	12,5	0	100	97,5	Home-CBP	78
Newborns Ush.	3,9±2.7	100	0	0	0	100	100	Home-CBP	78
Mother BA	14.4±8.7	28,5	46,5	12,5	12,5	87,5	52	Home-CBP	78
Mother Ush.	6.3±4.8	25	62,5	12,5	0	100	94	Home-CBP	78
6-23 months	27,1±11,5	3,6	27,5	42	26,9	73,1	16	Home-CBP	79
6-9ys.BA	20,2±1,3	14	41	28	17	83	38	Home-CBP	80
6-9ys.Ush	9,3±0,6	65	28	7	0	100	93	Home-CBP	80
6-9ys-Tuc	19,6±1,2	0	54,5	41,5	0	100	23	Home-CBP	80
24-52ys.BA	20,7±1,9	13	39	19	29	71	35	Home-CBP	81
Prem.summer	23,9±10,4	0	56	12,5	31,5	68,5	50	Diasorin	71,72
Prem.winter	13,8±5,3	25	69	6	0	100	62,5	Diasorin	71,72
Postm-summer	23,1±10,6	8	42	33	17	83	42	Diasorin	71,72
Postm.winter	14,2±7,2	18,5	75	6,5	0	100	75	Diasorin	71,72
Independent: 65-80ys.	17,9±0,6	11,5	49,6	29,5	9,4	90,6	85,4	IDS	53
Institutionalized:65-96ys.	13,6±6,1	32	54	14	0	100	100	Diasorin	84

c) Healthy Adults from 24 till 55ys. of Age

The nutritional status on Vitamin D was evaluated during winter time in 30 healthy young adults (12 men and 18 women) aged from 24 to 52ys. living in BA. The mean value of 25OHD was 20.7±1.9ng/ml without differences by gender. Deficiency was 13%; insufficiency 39%; hypovitaminosis 19% and adequacy 29% [81]. The clinical inadequacy was 71% while the DRI inadequacy was 35% (table 2).

A recent longitudinal research was conducted in pre (PM) and postmenopausal (M) women living in two southern cities of Argentina (Ushuaia: 54°S and Comodoro Rivadavia: 45°S) to evaluate the levels of 25OHD at the end of the winter vs. at the end of the summer. The results showed that the 25OHD levels were lower at the end of winter in both groups of women: PM (13.8±5.3 vs. 23.9±10.4, respectively; $p<0.05$) and M (14.2±7.2 vs. 23.1±10.6; $p<0.05$), without differences between them. A 25% and 18.5% of deficiency was observed in PM and M, respectively at the end of the winter while this percentage was lower (0% and 8% of PM and M, respectively) at the end of the summer. A 100% incidence of clinical inadequacy of vitamin D was observed in both groups at the end of winter while the inadequacy remained higher (69.5% and 83%, respectively) at the end of the summer [82-83]. The DRI inadequacy was 62.5% PM and 75%M at the end of the winter and 50% and 42% at the end of the summer (table 2).

d) Adults Older than 65 ys.

The aforementioned research conducted in Argentina by AAOMM in the healthy Argentinean population with an average of 71±5ys. also found a high incidence of clinical or DRI vitamin D inadequacy (91% and 80%, respectively). The mean value of 25OHD obtained in the 169 studied subjects was 17.9±0.64ng/ml. Severe vitamin D deficiency was in 11% of the subjects; insufficiency in 47%; hypovitaminosis in 33% and adequacy in 9% [53] (table 2).

e) Institutionalized Adults

The levels of 25OHD were comparatively evaluated in 97 institutionalized women aged from 65 to 96ys. living in similar social-status institutions and from two geographic cities which have a similar solar radiation index: Lleida (Spain) (n=49) and BA (Argentina) (n=48). The mean value of 25OHD was 11.7±5.8ng/ml in Lleida and 13.6±6.1ng/ml in BA. The analysis of the results evidenced a high prevalence of vitamin D deficiency/insufficiency even at the end of the summer. Deficiency was 47% in Lleida and 32% in BA; insufficiency 43% and 54%, respectively; hypovitaminosis 10% and 14%, respectively.

The clinical inadequacy was 100% in both cities while the DRI inadequacy was 94% in Lleida and 100% in BA (table 2).

2. Importance of Vitamin D Deficiency in Clinical and Pharmacological Interventions

A higher deficiency set point has important implications in therapeutic treatment because, according to clinical observations, the effectiveness of some anticatabolic drugs depends on the adequacy of vitamin D [85]. Regarding this, bisphosphonates are routinely prescribed for the treatment of postmenopausal osteoporosis. In clinical trials, these drugs have been found to increase BMD and to decrease fracture risk in the majority of the treated population.

An experimental research carried out in osteopenic rats presenting or not vitamin D insufficiency reliably evidenced the different response to the treatment with bisphosphonates [86]. Osteopenic vitamin D sufficient or insufficient rats, without sign of osteomalacia, were obtained by surgery and diet manipulation; then they were treated with the aminobisphosphonate olpadronate (Gador SA., Argentina) one a week during two remodeling cycles. A SHAM group received vitamin D throughout the study and was taken as control.

The bone volume at the end of the study and the change in the proximal tibia BMD between the end of the experiment and baseline demonstrated that the effectiveness of the anticatabolic treatment depended on the nutritional status of vitamin D (figures 3 and 4).

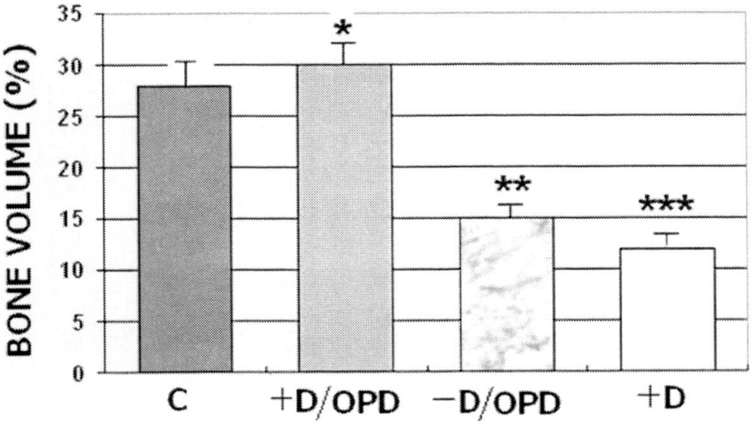

Figure 3. Bone volume (BV) (%) at the end of experiment. Data were expressed as mean ± SE. Untreated OVX rats (+D) presented a diminution in BV compared to C (p<0.001). OPD treatment prevented this decrease (**P < 0.01 compared to +D) and had a high effect in the +D group (*P <0.05 +D/OPD vs. −D/OPD).

Several clinical researches confirmed the negative interrelationship between bisphosphonate effectiveness and vitamin D inadequacy; however, the threshold of 25OHD levels for an optimal response differs among them. Ishijima M et al [87] reported that vitamin D status may affect the increase in lumbar spine BMD of postmenopausal Japanese osteoporotic women treated with 5mg/day of alendronate during 6 a month-period. The results suggested that a 25OHD level >25ng/ml appears to be required for an optimal response. Conversely, Adami et al [52] studied 1515 Italian women with postmenopausal osteoporosis under treatment with anti-resorbing agents during approximately 13 months. The results suggested that 25OHD levels above 50nmol/L or 20ng/ml seems to be necessary to maximize the response to anticatabolics, in terms of both BMD changes and anti-fracture efficacy.

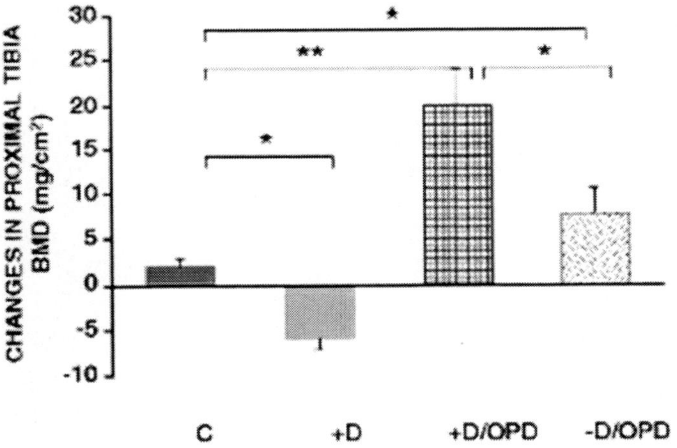

Figure 4. Percentage of change in proximal tibia BMD from baseline to the end of the experiment. Data were expressed as mean ± SE. Untreated rats (+D) exhibited lower BMD (*P<0.05) compared to C. OPD treatment prevented this decrease (**P < 0.01 compared to C) and had a high effect in the +D groups (*P <0.05 compared +D/OPD vs. −D/OPD).

Biochemical Assays of 25OHD

After 25OHD measurement was accepted as the best available marker of vitamin D nutritional status it has been widely used by clinicians to diagnose low vitamin D status, and subsequently to make decisions regarding supplementation or high-dose prescription of vitamin D. Although this analyte is highly stable in serum, a potentially large error or variability exists in the determination of 25OHD, so there is a large debate in the literature about how to accurately measure 25OHD [88-92].

The first method for measuring 25OHD was introduced in 1971 based on competitive protein binding after solvent extraction. Later, methods based on high performance liquid chromatography (HPLC) became available. The first radioimmunoassay (RIA) which incorporated a specific 25OHD antibody was developed in 1985. This method was partially, but no entirely, replaced by chemiluminescence (CLIA) or enzymatic (EIA) immunoassays. Nowadays, all this methods are in use.

Given the large number of methodologies available for the measurement of 25OHD, the choice of which is the best method for an individual laboratory is challenging especially for the dramatic increase of both routine clinical and research use of the measurement, over the last few years. Each method has advantages and limitations and differences remain between methodologies that confound the application of a single cut point (e.g., 30 ng/mL or 75 nmol/L) for the diagnosis of low vitamin D status [93]. Moreover, these commercial immunoassays show interassay CVs of ~10%, but it may be considerably higher (up to 25%) in the low range (e.g., <15nmol/L). This should be kept in mind when following an individual patient over time. Another problem is that although some assays may detect both metabolites to a similar degree, others may only detect vitamin D_3 metabolites [90]. This may lead to underestimation of the total 25OHD serum level.

Many tests have explored the differences in 25OHD levels in samples analyzed by using different assay types [88, 94-96]. In this regard, in 2004 Brinkley et al [89] alerted about the large variability in 25OHD result, both between methods and between laboratories and concluded that the measurement of 25OHD must be standardized. They compared the values reported from healthy individuals samples sent to six laboratories that used different methodologies and found a two-fold difference in the mean values that ranged from 42.8 to 89nmol/L (17.1–35.6ng/mL). This ample range demonstrated that for half of the samples, whether an individual was classified as having insufficient or normal vitamin D status, depended only on the laboratory used.

The last developed method introduced in 2004 was the liquid chromatography tandem mass spectroscopy (LC–MS/MS) which can measure the different vitamin D metabolites [98]. This very expensive technology, at least for countries such as Argentina and other developing countries, has improved 25OHD assay performance, thereby improving agreement between measurements obtained at different clinical laboratories. However, a review of recent vitamin D External Quality Assessment Scheme (DEQAS) data revealed substantial variability in individual 25OHD results between laboratories using such methodology. Interassay differences of 2.9 to 5.1ng/ml were also observed when the determination of 25OHD levels were compared by HPLC, LC-MS/MS, and RIA assays showing LC-MS/MS and RIA values higher than HPLC [99]. The conclusion that calibration did not eliminate interassay differences was suggested when the levels of 25OHD measured by LC-MS/MS was compared to the values of other seven commercially available assays [100]. The analytical uncertainties in measuring serum 25OHD was recently emphasized at the NIH workshop

''Nutrient Biomarkers Analytical Methodology: Vitamin D Workshop'' held on December 16, 2009 [100].

Assessing method comparability is not helped by the lack of a recommended reference method. A method based on gas chromatography mass spectrometry (GCMS) was developed [101]; however, its implementation as a reference method for the standardization of 25OHD was found to be extremely complex and was not widely used in assay development or in quality assurance programs [102]. The US National Institute of Standards and Technology (NIST) has very recently introduced serum based reference materials in four different concentrations covering the analytical range of 25OHD levels (SRM 972 NIH; http://www.nist.gov/cstl/analytical/organic/vitamindinserum.cfm) that enable the long term and worldwide standardization of 25OHD measurement.

Conclusion

Vitamin D inadequacy may have serious consequences for bone health and possibly for other non-skeletal tissues, both in children and in adults. The levels of 25OHD are the best index vitamin D nutritional status. Nowadays there is general consensus that 25OHD levels < 25nmol/l or 10ng/ml represent vitamin D deficiency; however, opinions vary on what should be an adequate serum 25OHD level. While clinicians consider a level near 75nmol/l or 30ng/ml as adequate, the American Committee which established the DRI for vitamin D assumes that this level is too high and that values between 40-50nmol/L or 16-20ng/ml are high enough to ensure bone health in most of the population with minimal sun exposure indicating that there is uncertainty about its extra-skeletal benefits; in addition, it suggested that a value of 70nmol/L or 28ng/ml for elderly people is associated with the lowest risk of hip fracture. Thus, one must be very careful when "normal" or even worse "deficient" vitamin D status with respect to circulating 25OHD is defined. The threshold level of 25OHD was obtained from population-based studies, and may differ between individuals depending on their age, skin colour, Ca intake or on their environmental situation (e.g. latitude, weather). Moreover, variability continues to exist in 25OHD assay methodology which would have an impact in the results. A reference method for the assay would be an optimal way to establish consensus on the required levels of serum 25OHD.

References

[1] Lips P. Vitamin D physiology. *Prog. Biophys. Mol. Biol. 2006;* 92:4-8.

[2] Strushkevich N, Usanov SA, Plotnikov AN, Jones G, Park HW. Structural analysis of CYP2R1 in complex with vitamin D3. *J. Mol. Biol. 2008;* 380:95-106.

[3] DeLuca HF. Overview of general physiologic features and functions of vitamin D. *Am. J. Clin. Nutr. 2004;* 80 (Suppl):1689S-96S.

[4] Holick MF. Vitamin D deficiency. *N. Engl. J. Med. 2007;* 357:266-81

[5] Holick MF. Photobiology of vitamin D. In: Feldman D, Pike JW, Glorieux FH, eds. *Vitamin D. 2nd ed. Burlington, MA: Elsevier Academic Press, 2005;*37-46.

[6] Department of Health Nutrition and bone health: with particular reference to calcium and vitamin D. *Report on Health and Social Subjects, 1998;49. London, United Kingdom: The Stationery Office.*

[7] Lips P. Vitamin D deficiency and secondary hyperparathyroidism in the elderly: consequences for bone loss and fractures and therapeutic implications. *Endocr. Rev. 2001;* 22:477-501.

[8] Ooms ME, Lips P, Roos JC, van der Vijgh WJ, Popp-Snijders C, Bezemer PD, et al. Vitamin D status and sex hormone binding globulin: determinants of bone turnover and bone mineral density in elderly women. *J. Bone Miner Res. 1995;* 10:1177-84.

[9] Brannon PM, Yetley EA, Bailey RL, Picciano MF. Overview of the conference "Vitamin D and health in the 21st century: an update. *Am. J. Clin. Nutr. 2008;* 88(Suppl):483S-90S.

[10] Nagpal S, Na S, Rathnachalam R. Noncalcemic actions of vitamin D receptor ligands. *Endocr. Rev. 2005;* 26:662-87.

[11] Bischoff-Ferrari HA, Dawson-Hughes B, Staehelin HB, Orav JE, Stuck AE, et al. Fall prevention with supplemental and active forms of vitamin D: a meta-analysis of randomised controlled trials. *BMJ 2009;* 339:b3692.

[12] Ginde AA, Mansbach JM, Camargo CA, Jr. Association between serum 25-hydroxyvitamin D level and upper respiratory tract infection in the Third National Health and Nutrition Examination Survey. *Arch. Intern. Med. 2009;* 169:384–90.

[13] Kim DH, Sabour S, Sagar UN, Adams S, Whellan DJ Prevalence of hypovitaminosis D in cardiovascular diseases (from the National Health and Nutrition Examination Survey 2001 to 2004). *Am. J. Cardiol. 2008;* 102:1540–44.

[14] Forman JP, Giovannucci E, Holmes MD, Bischoff-Ferrari HA, Tworoger SS, Willett WC, Curhan GC. Plasma 25-hydroxyvitamin D levels and risk of incident hypertension. *Hypertension 2007;* 49:1063–69.

[15] Hypponen E, Laara E, Reunanen A, Jarvelin MR, Virtanen SM. Intake of vitamin D and risk of type I diabetes: a birth-cohort study. *Lancet 2001;* 358:1500-03.

[16] Trump DL, Deeb KK, Johnson CS Vitamin D: considerations in the continued development as an agent for cancer prevention and therapy. *Cancer J. 2010;* 16:1–9.

[17] Brehm JM, Schuemann B, Fuhlbrigge AL, Hollis BW, Strunk RC, Zeiger RS, Weiss ST, Litonjua AA. Serum vitamin D levels and severe asthma exacerbations in the Childhood Asthma Management Program study. *J. Allergy Clin. Immunol. 2010;* 126:52-8.e5.

[18] Brehm JM, Celedon JC, Soto-Quiros ME, Avila L, Hunninghake GM, Forno E, Laskey D, Sylvia JS, Hollis BW, Weiss ST, Litonjua AA. Serum vitamin D levels and markers of severity of childhood asthma in Costa Rica. *Am. J. Respir. Crit. Care Med. 2009;* 179:765–771.

[19] Hollis BW. Circulating 25-Hidroxi D levels indicative of vitamin D sufficiency: implications for establishing a new effective dietary intake recommendation for vitamin D. *J. Nutr. 2005;* 135:317-22.

[20] Holick MF. Vitamin D: the underappreciated D-lightful hormone that is important for skeletal and cellular health. *Curr. Opin. Endocrinol. Diabetes 2002;* 9:87-98.

[21] Bacchetta J, Dubourg L, Harambat J, Ranchin B, Abou-Jaoude P, Arnaud S, Carlier MC, Richard M, Cochat P. The influence of glomerular filtration rate and age on

fibroblast growth factor 23 serum levels in pediatric chronic kidney disease. *J. Clin. Endocrinol. Metab. 2010*; 95:1741-8.

[22] Morris HA, Anderson PH. Autocrine and paracrine actions of vitamin D. *Clin. Biochem. Rev. 2010*; 31:129-38.

[23] Binkley N, Krueger DC, Morgan S, Wiebe S. Current status of clinical 25-hydroxyvitamin D measurement: An assessment of between-laboratory agreement. *Clinica Chimica Acta 2010*; 411:1976-82.

[24] Stamp TC, Haddad JG, Twigg CA. Comparison of oral 25-hydroxycholecalciferol, vitamin D, and ultraviolet light as determinants of circulating 25-hydroxyvitamin D. *Lancet 1977*; 1:1341-3.

[25] Norman AW, Bouillon R. Vitamin D nutritional policy needs a vision for the future. *Experim. Biol. Med. 2010*; 235:1034-45.

[26] Haddad JG, Chyu KJ. Competitive protein-binding radioassay for 25-hydroxycholecalciferol. *J. Clin. Endocrinol. Metab. 1971*; 33:992-5.

[27] Malabanan A, Veronikis IE, Holick MF. Redefining vitamin D insufficiency. *Lancet 1998*; 351:805-6.

[28] Eastwood JB, de Wardener HE, Gray RW, Lemann JL Jr. Plasma 1,25(OH)2 vitamin D concentrations in nutritional osteomalacia. *Lancet 1979*; 2:465.

[29] Need AG, O'Loughlin PD, Morris HA, Costes PS, Horowitz N, Nordin BE. Vitamin D metabolites and calcium absorption in severe vitamin D deficiency. *J. Bone Miner Res. 2008*; 23:1859-63.

[30] Mc Kenna MJ and Freaney R Secondary hyperparathyroidism in the elderly: means to defining hypovitaminosis D. *Osteoporosis Int. 1998;* 8(Suppl 2): 3-6.

[31] Lamberg-Allardt CJ, Outila TA, Kärkkainen MU, Rita HJ, Valsta LM. Vitamin D deficiency and bone health in healthy adults in Finland: could this be a concern in other parts of Europe? *J. Bone Miner Res. 2001;* 16:2066-73.

[32] Heaney RP. The vitamin D requirement in health and disease. *J. Steroid Biochem. Mol. Biol. 2005;* 97:13-9.

[33] Chapuy MC, Preziosi P, Maamer M, Arnaud S, Galan P, Hereberg S, Meunier PJ. Prevalence of vitamin D insufficiency in an adult normal population. *Osteoporosis Int. 1997;* 7:439-43.

[34] Steingrimsdottir L, Gunnarsson O, Indridason OS, Franzson L, Sigurdsson G. Relationship between serum parathyroid hormone levels, vitamin D sufficiency, and calcium intake. *JAMA 2005;* 294:2336-41.

[35] Bischoff-Ferrari HA, Giovannucci E, Willett WC, Dietrich T, Dawson-Hughes B. Estimation of optimal serum concentrations of 25-hydroxyvitamin D for multiple health outcomes. *Am. J. Clin. Nutr. 2006*; 84:18-28.

[36] Holick MF. Vitamin D status: measurement, interpretation, and clinical application. *Ann. Epidemiol. 2009*; 19:73-8.

[37] Dawson-Hughes B, Heaney RP, Holick MF, Lips P, Meunier PJ, Vieth R. Estimates of optimal vitamin D status. *Osteoporos Int. 2005*; 16:713-16.

[38] Need AG, O'Loughlin PD, Jesudason DR, Nordin BEC. Serum 25 hydroxyvitamin D level required to minimize bone resorption in postmenopausal women. *J. Bone Miner Res. 2002;* 17 (Suppl 1): S218.

[39] Heaney RP, Dowell MS, Hale CA, Bendich A. Calcium absorption varies within the reference range for serum 25-hydroxyvitamin D. *J. Am. Coll Nutr. 2003*;22:142– 6.

[40] Bischoff-Ferrari HA. How to select the doses of vitamin D in the management of osteoporosis. *Osteoporosis Int 2007*; 18:401-7.

[41] Melin AL, Wilske J, Ringertz H, Sääf M. Vitamin D status, parthyroid function and femoral bone density in an elderly Swedish population living at home. *Aging Clin. Exp. Res. 1999*; 11:200-7.

[42] Thomas MK, Lloyd-Jones DM, Thadani RI, Shaw AC, Deraska DJ, Kitch BT, Vamvakase C, Dick IM, Prince RL and Finkelstein JS. Hypovitaminosis D in medical inpatients. *N. Engl. J. Med. 1998;* 338:777-83.

[43] Chapuy MC, Arlot ME, Duboeuf F, Brun J, Crouzet B, Arnaud S, Delmas PD, Meunier PJ. Vitamin D3 and calcium to prevent hip fractures in the elderly women. *N. Engl. J. Med. 1992*; 327:1637-42.

[44] Lips P, Bouillon R, van Schoor NM, Vanderschueren D, Verschueren S, Kuchuk N, Milisen K, Boonen S. Reducing fracture risk with calcium and vitamin D. *Clin. Endocrinol. (Oxf) 2010*; 73:277-85.

[45] Gloth FM, Gunberg CM, Hollis BW, Haddad JG and Tobin JD. Vitamin D deficiency in homebound elderly persons. *JAMA 1995;*274,1683–6.

[46] Haden ST, Fuleihan GEH, Angell JE, Cotran NM, LeBoff MS. Calcidiol and PTH levels in women attending an osteoporosis Program. *Calcif Tissue Int 1999;*64:275-9.

[47] Dawson-Hughes B, Harris A, Krall E, Dallal G. Effect of calcium and vitamin D supplementation on bone density in men and women 65 years of age or older. *N. Eng. J. Med. 1997;* 337:670-6.

[48] Heaney RP, Armas LA, Shary JR, Bell NH, Binkley N, Hollis BW. 25-Hydroxylation of vitamin D3: relation to circulating vitamin D3 under various input conditions. *Am. J. Clin. Nutr. 2008;* 87:1738-42.

[49] Binkley N, Ramamurthy R, Krueger D. Low vitamin D status: definition, prevalence, consequences, and correction. *Endocrinol. Metab. Clin. North Am. 2010*; 39:287-301.

[50] Davies M, Heys SE, Selby PL, Berry JL, Mawer EB. Increased catabolism of 25-hydroxyvitamin D in patients with partial gastrectomy and elevated 1,25-dihydroxyvitamin D levels. Implications for metabolic bone disease. *J. Clin. Endocrinol. Metab. 1997;* 82:209-12.

[51] Clements MR, Johnson L, Fraser DR. A new mechanism for induced vitamin D deficiency in calcium deprivation. *Nature 1987*; 325:62-5.

[52] Adami S, Giannini S, Bianchi G, Sinigaglia L, Di Munno O, Fiore CE, Minisola S, Rossini M. Vitamin D status and response to treatment in post-menopausal osteoporosis. and response to treatment in post-menopausal osteoporosis. *Osteoporos Int. 2009*; 20:239-44.

[53] Oliveri B, Plantalech A, Bagur A, Wittich G, Rovai G, Pusiol E, Lopez Giovanelli J, Ponce G, Nieva A, Chaperon A, Ladizesky M, Somoza J, Casco C, Zeni SN, Parisi M y Mautalen C. High prevalence of vitamin D insufficiency in healthy elderly people living at home in Argentina. *Eur. J. Clin. Nutr. 2004;* 58:337-342.

[54] Plantalech L, Fassi J, PozzoMJ,Ercolano M,Ladizesky M, Casco C, Zeni S, Somoza J, Bagur A, Oliveri B: Hypovitaminosis D in elderly people living in an overpopulated city: Buenos Aires. In Focus in Nutrition Research. ED: Tony P. *Starks- Nova Science Publishers NY USA, 149-163, 2006.*

[55] Dietary References Intakes (DRI) for Calcium, Phosphorus, Magnesium, vitamin D and Fluoride. Standing Committee on the Scientific Evaluation of Dietary References

Intakes, Food and Nutrition Board and Institute of Medicine, National Academy of Sciences, Washington, D.C. 1997.

[56] Institute of Medicine of the National Academies. Dietary Reference Intakes for Calcium and Vitamin D. http://www.iom.edu/~/media/Files/ Report 2010. Dietary-Reference-Intakes-for-Calcium-and- Vitamin-D/Vitamin and Calcium 2010 Report Brief.pdf. Accessed Dec. 1, 2010.

[57] Russell RM Current framework for DRI development: what are the pros and cons? *Nutr. Rev. 2008*; 66:455-8.

[58] Institute of Medicine. The development of DRIs 1994–2004: lessons learned and new challenges-workshop summary. Washington, DC: The National Academies Press, *2008*.

[59] Cranney A, T. Horsley, S. O´Donnell, H.A. Weiler, L. puil, D.S. Ooi, s.A. Atkinson, L.M. Ward, D. Moher, D.A. Hanley, M. Fang, F. Yazdi, C. Garritty, M. Sampson, N. Barrowman, A. Tsertsvadze and V. Mamaladze. Effectiveness and safety of vitamin D in relation to bone health. Evidence Report/Technology Assessment, n°158 (Prepared by the University of Otawa Evidence-based Practice Center (UO-EPC) under contract n° 290-02-0021). AHRQ Publication n° 07-E013. Rockville, MD, Agency for Healthcare Research and Quality. 2007.

[60] Cranney A, Weiler HA, O'Donnell S, Puil L. Summary of evidence-based review on vitamin D efficacy and safety in relation to bone health. *Am. J. Clin. Nutr. 2008*;88:513S-9.

[61] Priemel M, von Domarus C, Klatte TO, Kessler S, Schlie J, Meier S, Proksch N, Pastor F, Netter C, Streichert T, Püschel K, Amling M. Bone mineralization defects and vitamin D deficiency: histomorphometric analysis of iliac crest bone biopsies and circulating 25-hydroxyvitamin D in 675 patients. *J. Bone Miner Res. 2010*; 25:305-12.

[62] Heaney RP, Holick MF. Why the IOM recommendations for vitamin D are deficient. *J. Bone Miner Res. 2011;*26:455-7.

[63] Reid IR, Avenell A. Evidence-based policy on dietary calcium and vitamin D. *J. Bone Miner Res. 2011*; 26:452-4.

[64] Heaney RP. Vitamin D: how much do we need, and how much is too much. *Osteoporois Int. 2000*; 11:553-5.

[65] Yetley EA. Assessing the vitamin D status of the US population. *Am. J. Clin Nut 2008;* 88: 558–64S.

[66] Prentice A. Vitamin D deficiency: a global perspective. *Nutr. Rev. 2008;* 66:S153-S64.

[67] Lewis JG, Elder PA. Serum 25-OH vitamin D2 and D3 are stable under exaggerated conditions. *Clin. Chem. 2008;* 54:1931-2.

[68] Binkley N, Novotny R, Krueger D, Kawahara T, Daida YG, Lensmeyer G, Hollis BW, Drezner MK. Low vitamin D status despite abundant sun exposure. *J. Clin. Endocrinol. Metab. 2007;* 92:2130-5.

[69] van der Mei IA, Ponsonby AL, Engelsen O, Pasco JA, McGrath JJ, Eyles DW, Blizzard L, Dwyer T, Lucas R, Jones G. The high prevalence of vitamin D insufficiency across Australian populations is only partly explained by season and latitude, *Environ. Health Perspect* 2007; 115:1132-39.

[70] Mansoor S, Habib A, Ghani F, Fatmi Z, Badruddin S, Mansoor S, Siddiqui I, Jabbar A. Prevalence and significance of vitamin D deficiency and insufficiency among apparently healthy adults. *Clin Biochem 2010*; 43:1431-5.

[71] Van der Wielen RPJ, Lowik MRH, van de Berg H, de Groot LCP, Haller J, Moreiras O, van Staveren WA. Vitamin D concentrations among elderly people in Europe. *Lancet 1995*; 346:207-210.

[72] Lips P, Ginkel van FC, Jongen MJM, Rubertus F, Vijgh van der WJF, Netelenbos JC. Determinants of vitamin D status in patients with hip fracture and in elderly control subjects. *Am. J. Clin. Nutr. 1987*; 46:1005-10.

[73] Lips P, Wiersinga A, van Ginkel FC, Jongen MJ, Netelenbos JC, Hackeng WH, Delmas PD, van der Vijgh WJ. The effect of vitamin D supplementation on vitamin D status and parathyroid function in elderly subjects. *J. Clin. Endocrinol. Metab. 1988*; 67:644-50.

[74] Holick MF. Vitamin D: a D-Lightful health perspective. *Nutr. Rev. 2008*; *66*:S182-94.

[75] Guillemant J, Taupin P, Le HT, Taright N, Allemanandou A, Pe´re`s G, et al. Vitamin D status during puberty in French health male adolescents. *Osteoporos Int. 1999*; 10:222-5.

[76] Melin A, Wilske J, Ringertz H, Sääf M. Seasonal variations in serum levels of 25-hydroxyvitamin D and parathyroid hormone but no detectable change in femoral neck bone density in an older population with regular outdoor exposure. *J. Am. Geriatr Soc. 2001*; 49:1190-6.

[77] Basile LA, Taylor SN, Wagner CL, et al. Neonatal vitamin D status at birth at latitude 32 degrees 72': evidence of deficiency. *J. Perinatol. 2007*; 27:568-71.

[78] Oliveri MB, Mautalen C, Alonso A, Velazquez H, Trouchot HA, Porto R, Martinez L and Barata AD. Estado nutricional de vitamina D en madres y neonatos de Ushuaia y Buenos Aires. *Medicina (Bs As) 1993*; 53:315-20.

[79] Duran P, Mangialavori G, Biglieri A, Kohan L, Aveya Gilardon E. Estudio descriptivo de la situación nutricional en niños de 6-72 meses de la República Argentina. Resultados de la Encuesta Nacional de Nutrición y Salud (ENNYS). *Arch. Argent. Pediatr.* 2009; 107:397-404.

[80] Oliveri MB, Ladizesky M, Sotelo A, Griffo S, Ballesteros G and Mautalen C (): Nutritional Rickets in Argentina. In *Nestlé Nutrition Workshops: Rickets* New York: Raven Press. *1991;* 21:233-224.

[81] Ladizesky M, Oliveri MB, Mautalen C. Niveles séricos de 25–hidroxi-vitamina D en la población normal de Buenos Aires. Su variación estacional. *Medicina (Buenos Aires) 1987;* 47:268-72.

[82] Pellegrini GG, Gonzales-Chaves MMS, Fajardo M, Ponce GM, Somoza J, Toyos GI, Zeni SN. Niveles de vitamina D en dos grupos de mujeres que habitan el sur argentino: efecto de la estación anual y su implicancia en el metabolismo óseo. *Actualizaciones en Osteologia 2009;* 5:103-4.

[83] Pellegrini GG, Gonzales-Chaves MMS, Fajardo M, Ponce GM, Toyos GI, Lifshitz F, Friedman S, Zeni SN. Salivary bone turnover markers in healthy pre and postmenopausal women: daily and seasonal rhythm. *Clin. Oral. Invest.* (in press).

[84] Portela ML, Mónico A, Barahona A, Dupraz H, Gonzales-Chaves MMS, Zeni SN. Comparative 25OH vitamin D levels in institutionalized women older than 65 years from two cities in Spain and Argentina. *USA. Nutrition 2011;* 26:283-9.

[85] Sebba AI. Significance of a decline in bone mineral density while receiving oral bisphosphonate treatment. *Clin. Ther. 2008*; 30:443-52.

[86] Mastaglia S, Pellegrini G, Mandalunis P, Gonzales Chaves M, Friedman S, Zeni SN. Vitamin D insufficiency reduces the protective effect of bisphosphonate on ovariectomy-induced bone loss in rats. *Bone 2006*; 39:837-44.

[87] Ishijima M, Sakamoto Y, Yamanaka M, Tokita A, Kitahara K, Kaneko H, Kurosawa H.Minimum required vitamin D level for optimal increase in bone mineral density with alendronate treatment in osteoporotic women. *Calcif Tissue Int 2009;* 85:398-404.

[88] Hollis BW. Editorial: The determination of circulating 25-hydroxyvitamin D: no easy task. *J. Clin. Endocrinol. Metab 2004;* 89:3149-51.

[89] Binkley N, Krueger D, Cowgill CS, Plum L, Lake E, et al. Assay variation confounds the diagnosis of hypovitaminosis D: a call for standardization. *J. Clin. Endocrinol. Metab. 2004*; 89:3152–7.

[90] Carter GD, Carter R, Jones J, Berry J. How accurate are assays for 25- hydroxyvitamin D? Data from the international vitamin D external quality assessment scheme. *Clin. Chem. 2004*; 50:2195-7.

[91] Glendenning P, Taranto M, Noble JM, Musk AA, Hammond C, Goldswain PR, Fraser WD, Vasikaran SD. Current assays overestimate 25-hydroxyvitamin D3 and underestimate 25-hydroxyvitamin D2 compared with HPLC: need for assay-specific decision limits and metabolite-specific assays. *Anal. Clin. Biochem. 2006*; 43:23-30.

[92] Zerwekh JE. The measurement of vitamin D: analytical aspects. *Anal. Clin. Biochem. 2004*; 41:272-81.

[93] Lips P, Chapuy MC, Dawson-Hughes B, Pols HA, Holick MF. An international comparison of serum 25-hydroxyvitamin D measurements. *Osteoporos Int. 1999*; 9:394-7.

[94] Binkley N, Krueger D, Lensmeyer G. 25-hydroxyvitamin D measurement, 2009: a review for clinicians. *J. Clin. Densitom. 2009*; 12:417-27.

[95] Lensmeyer GL, Wiebe DA, Binkley N, Drezner MK. HPLC method for 25-hydroxyvitamin D measurement: comparison with contemporary assays. *Clin. Chem. 2006*; 52:1120-6.

[96] Terry AH, Sandrock T, Meikle AW. Measurement of 25-hydroxyvitamin D by the Nichols ADVANTAGE, DiaSorin LIAISON, DiaSorin RIA, and liquid chromatography-tandem mass spectrometry. *Clin. Chem. 2005*; 51:1565-6.

[97] Chen H, McCoy LF, Schleicher RL, Pfeiffer CM. Measurement of 25-hydroxyvitamin D3 (25OHD3) and 25-hydroxyvitamin D2 (25OHD2) in human serum using liquid chromatography-tandem mass spectrometry and its comparison to a radioimmunoassay method. *Clin. Chim. Acta 2008;* 391:6-12.

[98] Vogeser M, Seger C, A decade of HPLC–MS/MS in the routine clinical laboratory—goals for further developments. *Clin. Biochem.* 2008; 41:649-62.

[99] van den Ouweland, JMW, Beijers AM, Demacker, PNM, van Daal H. Measurement of 25-OH-vitamin D in human serum using liquid chromatography tandem-mass spectrometry with comparison to radioimmunoassay and automated immunoassay. *J. Chromatography B: Analytical Technologies in the Biomedical and Life Sciences* 2010; 878:1163-1168.

[100] Binkley N, Krueger D, Lensmeyer G. 25-hydroxyvitamin D measurement, 2009: a review for clinicians. *J. Clin. Densitom. 2009*; 12:417-27.

[101] Carter GD. 25-Hydroxyvitamin D assays: the quest for accuracy. *Clin. Chem.* 2009; *55*:1300-2.

[102] Carter GD, Jones JC. Use of a common standard improves the performance of liquid chromatography-tandem mass spectrometry methods for serum 25- hydroxyvitamin-D. *Anal. Clin. Biochem. 2009*; 46:79-81.

[103] Vogeser M. Quantification of circulating 25-hydroxyvitamin D by liquid chromatography–tandem mass spectrometry. *J. Steroid Biochem. Mol. Biol.* 2010; 121:565-73.

In: Vitamin D Deficiency
Editors: V. Lerner and C. Miodownik
ISBN: 978-1-61470-964-0

Chapter II

Vitamin D Deficiency: An Independent Risk-Factor or a Marker of Poor Health

Yair Liel
Endocrine Unit, Soroka University Medical Center,
and the Faculty of Health Sciences, Ben-Gurion University of the Negev,
Beer-Sheva, Israel

Abstract

In the last few decades there has been much interest on extra-skeletal effects of vitamin D deficiency along with considerable expectations that vitamin D or its derivatives could provide new therapeutic approach to a wide variety of diseases. The most robust data on the beneficiary effects of vitamin D in extra-skeletal body systems derive from basic science and observational/epidemiological studies. Interventional studies are few and much less conclusive.

The current review provides an overview on the available data on extra-skeletal effects of vitamin D deficiency and available interventional studies, and presents the complexity of dissecting-out the role of vitamin D in given disease conditions. A paradigm is presented which attempts to reconcile between the impressive effects of vitamin D in extra-skeletal systems in basic research and epidemiological studies and the inconclusive results of the available controlled interventional studies. Available data support the notion that vitamin D deficiency is both an independent risk factor, and a non-specific marker of poor health.

In recent decades, skeletal and particularly extra-skeletal effects of vitamin D attracted significant scientific and public interest. Vitamin D deficiency became associated with a very wide variety of health disorders, which reminded of an index section of a medical textbook, and beyond (Table 1) [1].

The association of vitamin D deficiency with specific pathological condition implied that correction of vitamin D deficiency, or vitamin D treatment, could possibly provide beneficial outcomes in those medical conditions. Subsequently, recommendations for target serum concentrations of 25-hydroxyvitamin D [25 (OH) D] increased, which were higher than previously recommended levels, and much higher doses of vitamin D were required to achieve those levels, exceeding most of the recommended daily allowances (RDA) issued by health authorities.

It wasn't until recently that the glorification of vitamin D has reached a point in which an inevitable question aroused: "The miracle of vitamin D: Sound science or hype?" (New-York Times, February 1, 2010). The issue reached the scientific and public arena largely as a due to an anticipation to the Institute of Medicine's extensive report on vitamin D, which when finally published ended up concluding that for most extra-skeletal effects, including cancer, falls, cardio-vascular, metabolic and autoimmune disorders, evidence for beneficial effects of vitamin D was inconclusive [2, 3].

The present review aims to follow landmarks in the development of the "vitamin D myth" that relate to its extra-skeletal effects, to delineate some of the known and the less appreciated facts regarding the role of vitamin D as a health modulator, and propose an alternative perspective for the role of vitamin D deficiency and sufficiency in health maintenance.

Landmarks in the History of Vitamin D

The first know description of osteomalacia is attributed to Francis Glisson as early as 1650.

However, the condition reached epidemic proportions in the 19th century, coincidental with the industrial revolution that was associated with massive air pollution, urbanization, and widespread child labor. Children's labor conditions deprived them of the limited sunlight that penetrated the prevalent heavy smog. Observations throughout the 19th century and the beginning of the 20th century contributed to the understanding of the link between sunlight and osteomalacia, the salutary influence of sunlight and fish-oil on osteomalacia, culminating about 1936 with the chemical characterization of vitamin D [4, 5].

The full activation sequence of vitamin D was elucidated in the early 1970s, with the discovery of 1,25-dihydroxyvitamin D [1,25$(OH)_2$D], the active metabolite of vitamin D, by DeLuca et al. [6]. The initial notion was that the biosynthesis of 1,25$(OH)_2$D, the final activation step of vitamin D, occurred exclusively in the kidneys as part of a specific endocrine system, , that included parathyroid hormone (PTH) and hypophosphatemia as the main stimuli of 1,25$(OH)_2$D synthesis, aimed at maintaining stable concentration of extracellular ionized calcium.

Table 1. Health conditions associated with vitamin D deficiency

Musculoskeletal
Bone health (osteoporosis, rickets, osteomalacia)
Falls in the elderly
Rehabilitation rates
Back pain in elderly women
Primary hyperparathyroidism bone disease
hypocalcemia after parathyroidectomy
Metabolic
Diabetes mellitus
Mortality: total and cardiovascular
Cancer incidence and mortality
Immune diseases
Multiple sclerosis
Inflammatory bowel disease
Bronchial asthm
Allergic rhinitis
SLE
Rheumatoid arthritis
Infectious diseases
Tuberculosis
influenza and URI
Periodontal diseases
HIV infection- AIDS
Obstetric complications
Pre-eclampsia
Cesarean section
Miscellaneous
Psoriasis
Mental illnesses
Cognitive function
Coagulation and thrombosis
Age-related macular degeneration

Mechanism of Action of Vitamin D

$1,25(OH)_2D$, the most active metabolite of vitamin D mediates its biological action through binding to specific cytosolic receptors (VDR), which act as transcription factors that control the synthesis of a variety of proteins, e.g.: enzymes, calcium channels, bone matrix proteins, and mediators of cell proliferation and differentiation. The discovery of VDR evolved throughout the 1970s, mainly through the pioneering work of Haussler and Norman [7], followed by purification and DNA sequencing in the 1980s. VDR were initially identified in intestinal tissues, but they were soon found in a wide variety of other tissues and cells, including such that are not involved in mineral or bone metabolism (Table 2).

Table 2. Tissues and cells distribution of vitamin D receptors (VDR)

GI tract
Parathyroid
Skeletal muscles *
Skin
Osteoblasts
Pancreatic β-cells
T and B-lymphocytes
Mononuclear cells
Myocardium *
Blood vessels
Vascular smooth muscles
Endothelial cells
Breast
Brain,
Pituitary
Gonads
Prostate

* According to Wang and DeLuca (Endocrinology 152:354, 2011) the ascription of VDR in skeletal and myocardial muscles was erroneous.

Table 3. Tissues and cells distribution of 25-hydroxyvitamin D-1α-hydroxylase

Kidney
Monocytes/Macrophages
lymphocytes
Skin
keratinocytes
Placenta
Blood vessels
Vascular smooth muscle
Endothelial cells
Brain
Prostate
Pancreatic islands
Osteoblasts
Parathyroid
Adrenal medulla
Colon
Adipocytes
Pancreatic islets
Neoplastic cells

In the early 1980s, following the recognition of the role of $1,25(OH)_2D$ in the pathogenesis of hypercalcemia in sarcoidosis and other granulomatous diseases, it became evident that macrophages contained 25-hydroxyvitamin D-1α-hydroxylase [1α -hydroxylase], the key enzyme for activation of vitamin D, that control of 1,25$(OH)_2$D synthesis in macrophages was unlike and different from the mechanism controlling 1,25$(OH)_2$D in the kidneys, and was particularly dissociated from physiological stimuli related to calcium homeostasis. 1α-hydroxylase was subsequently identified in a variety of cells and tissues (table 3). The widespread distribution of VDR and 1α-hydroxylase, often in the same tissues, brought about the notion that vitamin D could carry specific roles in different tissues and that its action in those tissues is carried-out by autocrine/paracrine mechanisms and controlled by tissue-specific mechanisms.

Extra-Skeletal ("Non-Classical") Effects of Vitamin D

Even though an extensive review of the extra-skeletal effects of vitamin D is beyond the scope of this review, short summaries of the main extra-skeletal effects of vitamin D will be presented to demonstrate the complexity of the positioning of vitamin D in the framework of the pathogenesis of various conditions.

Vitamin D, Muscle Strength and Falls

There seems to be a wide agreement that vitamin D is an effective means of preventing falls in the elderly [8]. It should be noted, however, that administration of mega-doses of vitamin D increased the risk of falls and fractures [9]. A recently published study even challenged the mere existence of VDR in skeletal muscle cells [10], casting doubt on the premise that the effect of vitamin D on muscles is mediated through VDR. Alternative mechanisms of action could be through effects on neurons and calcium and phosphorus homeostasis.

Vitamin D and Cardiovascular Morbidity

Vitamin D was ascribed an important role in preventing cardiovascular morbidity and mortality [11, 12]. Basic studies revealed significant effects of vitamin D on suppression of the renin-angiotensin axis activity and other specific effects on vascular walls [13, 14]. Mice devoid of vitamin D present increased activity of the renin-angiotensin axis, increased pro-inflammatory cytokines activity, decreased activity anti- inflammatory cytokines activity, hypercoagulability, decreased fibrinolytic activity, hypertension, myocardial hypertrophy and fibrosis and heart failure, suggesting a protective cardiovascular influence of vitamin D activity [13]. It should be noted that in different models vitamin D itself could increase vascular calcification [15].

Most available studies related to cardiovascular effects of vitamin D (peripheral vascular disease and myocardial infarction) are observational. The extent of vitamin D deficiency in the patients' groups and the differences between patients and controls were also small enough to raise doubt regarding their biological significance. [12, 16].

Studies, which examined the effect of vitamin D or its active metabolites on blood pressure in human's revealed fairly consistent beneficial effects, mainly on diastolic blood pressure. The findings were of borderline statistical significance, and the mean differences between treatment and control groups was of the order of 3-4 mmHg [17, 18].

Several studies addressed the role of vitamin D in heart failure. Out of eight studies that examined the relationship between heart failure and vitamin D, seven were observational and indicated a direct relationship between vitamin D deficiency morbidity and survivability from heart failure. In the only interventional study, there was no difference in survival between the placebo and vitamin D-treated group [12].

An ultimate answer for the clinical impact of vitamin D on the cardiovascular system is expected to emerge from results of the "VITAL" study, a controlled intervention trial sponsored by the U.S. Institutes of Health (NIH), an ongoing study aimed to examines the long-term effects of 2000 units per day of vitamin D, omega 3, or both, on morbidity and mortality from cardiovascular and cancer [19].

Vitamin D and Type-2 Diabetes Mellitus

Basic studies provide evidence suggesting beneficial effects of vitamin D on carbohydrate metabolism. $1,25(OH)_2D$ was shown to increases insulin secretion by pancreatic islet-cells, directly through binding to the insulin-gene promoter region, and indirectly as a result of increased synthesis of osteocalcin and by maintaining the calcium homeostasis. $1,25(OH)_2D$ was also shown to increase insulin sensitivity by increasing the expression of insulin receptor in peripheral tissues and activation of PPAR-δ [20].

Observational studies revealed a consistent inverse association between vitamin D levels and the incidence of type-2 diabetes [20, 21]. On the other hand, results of interventional studies were less certain. While some studies demonstrated an increased sensitivity to insulin, there was no demonstrable effect on fasting glucose, which consisted the main goal of those studies [20].

Vitamin D and the Immune System

Heliotherapy remained an acceptable means of treatment in patients with tuberculosis, at least until the mid 20th century. Its possible mechanism of action included the synthesis of vitamin D, by the influence of solar radiation, final activation of vitamin D in the kidneys and in active granulomas sites. $1,25(OH)_2D$ could stimulate the secretion of anti-microbial proteins acting on biological membranes enabling the killing bacteria, viruses and fungi, and at the same time increasing the ability of eradication of intracellular bacteria, such as in the case of tuberculosis [22].

Three studies that examined the effect of vitamin D on the rate of recovery in patients with tuberculosis treated with conventional anti-tuberculosis drugs did not reveal modest to nil results [23-25]. In one of the studies the clearance rate of acid-fast bacteria from sputum smears was somewhat faster in the initial 6 weeks of treatment in the vitamin D-treated group [24]. In the other 2 studies vitamin D treatment produced no overall effect, except one of those studies in which shortening of the sputum culture recovery time was observed, but only in patients carrying a specific genotypes of VDR [23].

Despite the multiple beneficial effects attributed to vitamin D including the metabolic system, muscle strength and microbial killing, no relationship could be demonstrated between vitamin D levels and neither length of hospitalization nor mortality in a mixed population of critically ill patients, including a subgroup of septic patients [26].

Vitamin D and Autoimmune Diseases

Basic studies have shown that Vitamin D has moderating effect on immune and inflammatory processes [27]. Epidemiological studies have suggested an inverse association between serum vitamin D levels and autoimmune diseases, such as systemic lupus erythematosus (SLE), rheumatoid arthritis, multiple sclerosis, inflammatory bowel diseases and diabetes mellitus type-1. A review of observational studies and case-control studies of vitamin D treatment in children suggested that vitamin D supplementation could decrease the rate of development of type-1 diabetes [28]. However, in the absence of randomized controlled studies, the clinical significance and applicability of those findings is unclear.

Vitamin D and Cancer

Following the discovery of VDR in cancer cells and observations indicating inhibitory effect of $1,25(OH)_2D$ on cell proliferation as well as pro-differentiative effect, there were considerable expectations concerning the clinical use of vitamin D or its derivatives in prevention and treatment of cancer [29].

Epidemiological studies indicate an inverse relation between sun exposure and levels of vitamin D on the one hand, and incidence rates of various malignant diseases on the other hand [23]. The few available interventional studies do not support a significant role for vitamin D in prevention of cancer [30].

In addition to its examination of metabolic and cardiovascular aspects, the ongoing NIH-supported “VITAL” study (see above), is also intended to address the cancer preventing properties of vitamin D.

The Complexity of Assessing the Role of Vitamin D Deficiency in Extra-Skeletal Morbidity

There are considerable difficulties in decoding the relationship between actual levels of vitamin D, or indirect accepted markers of vitamin D levels (such as decreased sunlight exposure or residence at higher geographical latitude) and extra-skeletal morbidity.

A major difficulty lies in the fact that vitamin D blood level does not reliably reflect its biological activity. Many of the different definitions of optimal level of vitamin D are based on the existence of an inverse correlation between the concentration of 25(OH)D and PTH concentration in blood. However, while there is no basic disagreement regarding the existence of such relationship, one cannot ignore the wide dispersion of the PTH around the regression curve, particularly at low concentrations of vitamin D [31]. It should be noted that 25(OH)D, which provides the best reflection on vitamin D stores is not by itself the biologically active metabolite of vitamin D and that the serum concentration of $1,25(OH)_2D$, the biologically active metabolite, is maintained at constant levels even at considerably low serum levels of 25(OH)D. Moreover, activation of vitamin D is differently controlled in the kidneys and extra-skeletal tissues. Factors such as age, renal function, blood concentration of vitamin D-binding protein (DBP) [32], ethnic descent and different VDR genotypes are some of the variables that may affect the biological activity of vitamin D. Finally, bad health itself may avert patients from sunlight exposure and block endogenous vitamin D synthesis.

Certain confounders could distort the perception regarding the role of vitamin D and extra-skeletal morbidity: 1. An inverse correlation exists between body mass and vitamin D levels, whereas body mass is directly correlated with a wide range of morbidities (metabolic, cardiovascular and malignant). 2. A direct association exists between engagement in physical activity and level of vitamin D, while there are health effects of physical activity that may be independent of vitamin D [33]. 3. Certain drugs could affect vitamin D levels. 4. While some observational studies assume that there is an inverse correlation between geographical latitude and levels of vitamin D, at least some U.S. and European studies reveal lack of such association and even a direct correlation between geographical latitude and levels of vitamin D (higher vitamin D level with higher latitudes) [34, 35]. 5. Urban air pollution, a well-recognized cause of a wide range of morbidity in itself, adversely affects the level of vitamin D [36]. 6. Socio-economic situation might adversely affect both general health condition and level of vitamin D [35].

The following proposed scenario considers low socio-economic condition as the lowest common denominator for increased morbidity and vitamin D deficiency (figure 1): Low socio-economic condition is by itself a known determinant of poor health [37].

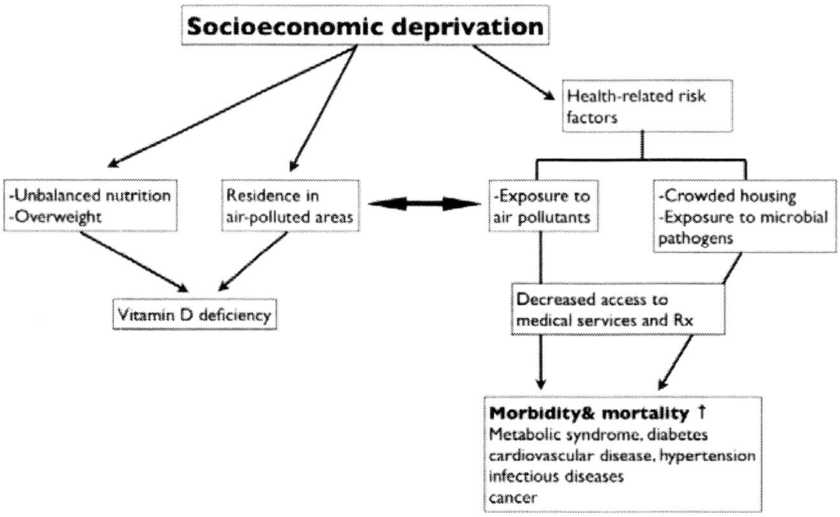

Figure 1.

Indigent populations often live in air-polluted cities, in crowded housing conditions, suffer from unbalanced nutrition and have a tendency for overweight [38]. Environmental pollution, overcrowding, and excess weight are known risk factors for increased morbidity aggravated by inadequate access to health services. Poor diet, excess weight and air pollution are also recognized risk factors for vitamin D deficiency. Thus, this scenario sets vitamin D deficiency in context with other risk factors and emphasizes the need to neutralize such factors in any attempt to assess the net role of vitamin D as a significant contributor to extra-skeletal morbidity.

Conclusion

Despite a remarkable range of biological activities demonstrated in well-defined controlled laboratory settings, and a large number of epidemiological observations linking vitamin D deficiency with a wide variety of extra-skeletal diseases, the results of interventional, controlled studies are hesitant and far less robust. This disparity could be due to the fact that laboratory studies may represent narrow aspects of the effect of vitamin D on defined systems, often simulating extreme conditions that do not necessarily reflect complex physiological and clinical situations. Some observational studies were biased due to failure to control for known confounders (let alone hidden confounders).

The reservations cast in this review are not intended to disprove the existence of a contributing role for vitamin D in health maintenance and treatment of extra-skeletal diseases, but rather to demonstrate the reciprocal relationship of vitamin D with other risk factors. Hopefully, future well-designed, randomized controlled studies, such as the ongoing "VITAL" study, could provide clearer perspective of the extra-skeletal health maintaining capabilities of vitamin D. Until further data is obtained, it seems prudent to conclude that vitamin D deficiency is both an independent risk factor, at least for some extra-skeletal diseases and a non-specific marker of poor health.

References

[1] Holick MF: Vitamin D: extraskeletal health. *Endocrinol. Metab. Clin. North Am.* 39:381-400, 2010.

[2] Ross CA, Taylor CL, Yaktine AL et al.: Committee to review dietary reference intakes for vitamin D and calcium food and nutrition board. Dietary reference intakes for calcium and vitamn D. 2010.

[3] Ross AC, Manson JE, Abrams SA et al.: The 2011 report on dietary reference intakes for calcium and vitamin D from the Institute of Medicine: what clinicians need to know. *J. Clin. Endocrinol. Metab.* 96:53-58, 2011.

[4] DeLuca HF: Evolution of our understanding of vitamin D. *Nutr. Rev.* 66:S73-87, 2008.

[5] Wolf G: The discovery of vitamin D: the contribution of Adolf Windaus. *J. Nutr.* 134:1299-1302, 2004.

[6] Holick MF, Schnoes HK, DeLuca HF: Identification of 1,25-dihydroxycholecalciferol, a form of vitamin D3 metabolically active in the intestine. *Proc. Natl. Acad. Sci. USA* 68:803-804, 1971.

[7] Haussler MR, Myrtle JF, Norman AW: The association of a metabolite of vitamin D3 with intestinal mucosa chromatin in vivo. *J. Biol. Chem.* 243:4055-4064, 1968.

[8] Cameron ID, Murray GR, Gillespie LD et al.: Interventions for preventing falls in older people in nursing care facilities and hospitals. *Cochrane Database Syst. Rev.* CD005465, 2010.

[9] Sanders KM, Stuart AL, Williamson EJ et al.: Annual high-dose oral vitamin D and falls and fractures in older women: a randomized controlled trial. *JAMA* 303:1815-1822, 2010.

[10] Wang Y, DeLuca HF: Is the vitamin d receptor found in muscle? *Endocrinology* 152:354-363, 2011.

[11] Dobnig H, Pilz S, Scharnagl H et al.: Independent association of low serum 25-hydroxyvitamin D and 1,25-dihydroxyvitamin D levels with all-cause and cardiovascular mortality. *Arch. Intern Med.* 168:1340-1349, 2008.

[12] Nemerovski CW, Dorsch MP, Simpson RU et al.: Vitamin D and cardiovascular disease. *Pharmacotherapy* 29:691-708, 2009.

[13] Li YC, Kong J, Wei M et al.: 1,25-Dihydroxyvitamin D(3) is a negative endocrine regulator of the renin-angiotensin system. *J. Clin. Invest.* 110:229-238, 2002.

[14] Somjen D, Weisman Y, Kohen F et al.: 25-hydroxyvitamin D3-1alpha-hydroxylase is expressed in human vascular smooth muscle cells and is upregulated by parathyroid hormone and estrogenic compounds. *Circulation* 111:1666-1671, 2005.

[15] Zebger-Gong H, Muller D, Diercke M et al.: 1,25-Dihydroxyvitamin D3-induced aortic calcifications in experimental uremia: up-regulation of osteoblast markers, calcium-transporting proteins and osterix. *J. Hypertens* 29:339-348, 2011.

[16] Manson JE, Allison MA, Carr JJ et al.: Calcium/vitamin D supplementation and coronary artery calcification in the Women's Health Initiative. *Menopause* 17:683-691, 2010.

[17] Burgaz A, Orsini N, Larsson SC et al.: Blood 25-hydroxyvitamin D concentration and hypertension: a meta-analysis. *J. Hypertens* 29:636-645, 2011.

[18] Witham MD, Nadir MA, Struthers AD: Effect of vitamin D on blood pressure: a systematic review and meta-analysis. *J. Hypertens* 27:1948-1954, 2009.

[19] Manson JE: Vitamin D and the heart: why we need large-scale clinical trials. *Cleve Clin. J. Med.* 77:903-910, 2010.

[20] Pittas AG, Lau J, Hu FB et al.: The role of vitamin D and calcium in type 2 diabetes. A systematic review and meta-analysis. *J. Clin. Endocrinol. Metab.* 92:2017-2029, 2007.

[21] Pittas AG, Sun Q, Manson JE et al.: Plasma 25-hydroxyvitamin D concentration and risk of incident type 2 diabetes in women. *Diabetes Care* 33:2021-2023, 2010.

[22] White JH: Vitamin D signaling, infectious diseases, and regulation of innate immunity. *Infect. Immun.* 76:3837-3843, 2008.

[23] Martineau AR, Timms PM, Bothamley GH et al.: High-dose vitamin D(3) during intensive-phase antimicrobial treatment of pulmonary tuberculosis: a double-blind randomised controlled trial. *Lancet* 377:242-250, 2011.

[24] Nursyam EW, Amin Z, Rumende CM: The effect of vitamin D as supplementary treatment in patients with moderately advanced pulmonary tuberculous lesion. *Acta. Med. Indones* 38:3-5, 2006.

[25] Wejse C, Gomes VF, Rabna P et al.: Vitamin D as supplementary treatment for tuberculosis: a double-blind, randomized, placebo-controlled trial. *Am. J. Respir. Crit. Care Med.* 179:843-850, 2009.

[26] Lucidarme O, Messai E, Mazzoni T et al.: Incidence and risk factors of vitamin D deficiency in critically ill patients: results from a prospective observational study. *Intensive Care Med.* 36:1609-1611, 2010.

[27] Bikle D: Nonclassic actions of vitamin D. *J. Clin. Endocrinol. Metab.* 94:26-34, 2009.

[28] Zipitis CS, Akobeng AK: Vitamin D supplementation in early childhood and risk of type 1 diabetes: a systematic review and meta-analysis. *Arch. Dis. Child* 93:512-517, 2008.

[29] Ingraham BA, Bragdon B, Nohe A: Molecular basis of the potential of vitamin D to prevent cancer. *Curr. Med. Res. Opin.* 24:139-149, 2008.

[30] Manson JE, Mayne ST, Clinton SK: Vitamin D and Prevention of Cancer - Ready for Prime Time? *N. Engl. J. Med.* 2011.

[31] Vieth R, Ladak Y, Walfish PG: Age-related changes in the 25-hydroxyvitamin D versus parathyroid hormone relationship suggest a different reason why older adults require more vitamin D. *J. Clin. Endocrinol. Metab.* 88:185-191, 2003.

[32] Thrailkill KM, Jo CH, Cockrell GE et al.: Enhanced excretion of vitamin D binding protein in type 1 diabetes: a role in vitamin D deficiency? *J. Clin. Endocrinol. Metab.* 96:142-149, 2011.

[33] McCullough ML, Weinstein SJ, Freedman DM et al.: Correlates of circulating 25-hydroxyvitamin D: Cohort Consortium Vitamin D Pooling Project of Rarer Cancers. *Am. J. Epidemiol.* 172:21-35, 2010.

[34] Holick MF, Siris ES, Binkley N et al.: Prevalence of Vitamin D inadequacy among postmenopausal North American women receiving osteoporosis therapy. *J. Clin. Endocrinol. Metab.* 90:3215-3224, 2005.

[35] Kuchuk NO, van Schoor NM, Pluijm SM et al.: Vitamin D status, parathyroid function, bone turnover, and BMD in postmenopausal women with osteoporosis: global perspective. *J. Bone Miner Res.* 24:693-701, 2009.

[36] Manicourt DH, Devogelaer JP: Urban tropospheric ozone increases the prevalence of vitamin D deficiency among Belgian postmenopausal women with outdoor activities during summer. *J. Clin. Endocrinol. Metab.* 93:3893-3899, 2008.

[37] Nelson K, Taylor L, Lurie N et al.: Neighborhood Environment and Health Status and Mortality Among Veterans. *J. Gen. Intern. Med.* 2011.

[38] James WP, Nelson M, Ralph A et al.: Socioeconomic determinants of health. The contribution of nutrition to inequalities in health. *BMJ* 314:1545-1549, 1997.

In: Vitamin D Deficiency
Editors: V. Lerner and C. Miodownik
ISBN: 978-1-61470-964-0

Chapter III

Vitamin D and Hypertension

José-Luis Pérez-Castrillón[1]* and Marta Ruiz-Mambrilla[2]
[1]Río Hortega University Hospital, Endocrinology Institute, Valladolid, Spain
[2]Rehabilitation and Language Medical Centre, Valladolid, Spain

Abstract

Adequate vitamin D levels are necessary for good vascular health. Vitamin D, in addition to increasing intestinal calcium absorption, reducing parathyroid hormone levels and improving the amount and quality of bone, has a beneficial vascular effect. Vitamin D deficiency has been associated with arterial hypertension. The association between hypertension and vitamin D deficiency is mediated by activation of the renin-angiotensin-aldosterone system. High calcitriol levels reduce plasma renin activity, leading to reduced plasma angiotensin II levels. This modulation of the renin-angiotensin-aldosterone system, besides reducing blood pressure, decreases inflammation in the vascular endothelium, limiting the progression of atherosclerosis. The objective of this review is to evaluate the possible relationship between hypertension and vitamin D.

Keywords: Vitamin D, Hypertension

Abbreviations

ABMP	Ambulatory blood-pressure monitoring
BMI	Body Mass Index
BP	Blood Pressure
CI	Confidence Interval
EVOS-	European Vertebral Osteoporosis Study

* Correspondence author: Jose Luis Pérez Castrillon, MD,PhD, Associate Professor of Medicine, Río Hortega University Hospital, Endocrinology Institute, Valladolid, Spain, C/Dulzaina, 2, 47016 Valladolid, E-mail: castrv@terra.es.

IL-	Interleukin
IOM-NAS -	Institute of Medicine-National Academy of Science
LASA-	Longitudinal Aging Study Amsterdam
NHNES III-	Third National Health and Nutrition Examination Survey
NF-KB	Nuclear Factor Kappa B
OR	Odds ratio
PTH	Parathyroid Hormone
RAAS-	Renin-Angiotensin-Aldosterone System
TNF	Tumoral Necrosis Factor
VDR-RXR-	itamin D Receptor- Receptor –X- Retinoid
WHI-	Women's Health Initiative

Introduction

Vitamin D has passed from simply being considered as an anti-rickets factor to be classified firstly as a vitamin and subsequently as an endocrine system that plays a key role in the regulation of the phospho-calcium metabolism. Although this role is, perhaps, the best known, vitamin D also plays a role in other actions such as modulation of the immune response, cell differentiation, and the prevention of diseases such as type I diabetes, tumors and dermatological diseases such as psoriasis [1]. It also plays a role in the prevention and development of cardiovascular diseases such as hypertension and heart failure [2].

Vitamin D comes from two main sources: the diet and cutaneous synthesis of ultraviolet B light. In the bloodstream it binds with 25-hydroxyvitamin D binding protein, the specific transport protein, and undergoes various metabolic activating processes. The first occurs in the liver and involves hydroxylation at position 25, resulting in 25-hydroxycholecalciferol (calcidiol).This metabolite is the main indicator of vitamin D levels in the body due to its elevated half life and because levels are directly related to the substrate level without being subjected to enzymatic regulation. Later there is a second hydroxylation in the kidney at position 1-α, giving rise to 1.25-dihydroxycholecalciferol (calcitriol), the active metabolite. To exert its effect it bonds with and causes a conformational change in the vitamin D receptor, and bonds with the retinoid X receptor to form a heterodimer, VDR-RXR. This structure penetrates the nucleus, where it inhibits or stimulates various genes, including two that may be important in cardiovascular disease; the TNF system activating protein, which regulates inflammatory cytokines, and the c-myc gene, which regulates cell proliferation and differentiation [3].There is another, non-genomic action, that uses the entrance of calcium into the muscle fibre through the calcium channels [1].

Vitamin D, in addition to increasing intestinal absorption of calcium, reducing levels of the parathyroid hormone (PTH levels) and improving the quantity and quality of bone, has a beneficial vascular effect. An association between vitamin D deficiency and peripheral arterial disease and myocardial infarction has been reported [4,5].

Levels of Vitamin D

Currently, several laboratory techniques permit measurement of the different metabolites of vitamin D. Of these, 25-hydroxycholecalciferol is the most appropriate metabolite for measuring vitamin D deposits. This has been accepted since 1997 by the panel on calcium and related nutrients of the food and nutrition board of the Institute of Medicine-National Academy of Sciences (IOM-NAS). There are two reasons. First, the long half-life of 25-hydroxycholecalciferol, three weeks, which reflects the production of vitamin D derived from cutaneous synthesis due to ultraviolet radiation and, to a lesser extent, from the diet. Second, the hepatic production of 25-hydroxycholecalciferol depends on the level of substrate, and is not regulated by enzymes. There are various methods of determination, with high-performance liquid chromatography (HPLC) being the method of choice, but the most-frequently used methods are chemoimmunoluminescence or enzyme immunoassay [6].

Levels of vitamin D can be classified as deficient (25-hydroxycholecalciferol <30nmol / l), insufficient (25-hydroxycholecalciferol 30 nml-50 nmol/L) and normal (25-hydroxycholecalciferol <50 nmol/L) [7]. Using these values as a reference, a high prevalence of vitamin D deficiency has been observed worldwide. A recently study, using data from the National Health and Nutrition Examination Survey, determined vitamin D levels in 4495 subjects and found a rate of vitamin D deficiency of 41.6%, with a higher rate in Hispanics (69%) and blacks (82%). These data come from the general population and were higher in the elderly and hospitalized subjects [8]. In a study conducted in Spain that included 451 people aged 65 years or more, the results showed a prevalence of vitamin D deficiency of 79% in non-hospitalized subjects compared to 91% in hospitalized individuals [9]. Similar results were found by Quesada et al [10] in Cordoba (Spain), which is located below parallel 40. This study analyzed 114 elderly patients with a mean age of 77 years, and found that 100% of institutionalized patients and 68% of outpatients had insufficient vitamin D levels. The cut-off point for measuring vitamin D insufficiency was 37.5 nmol/L.

Gomez Alonso et al [11] studied 326 younger individuals from the European Vertebral Osteoporosis Study (EVOS) cohort and found vitamin D deficiency in 27% of cases and insufficiency (25-hydroxycholecalciferol <45 nmol/L) in 45% of cases.

Taken together, these data show the high prevalence of vitamin D deficiency and insufficiency. This constitutes a major public health problem and may be a prevalent vascular risk factor.

Epidemiology

Cardiovascular diseases are the most common cause of mortality and morbidity in developed countries. An increasing number of risk factors are now thought to be involved. There is ample evidence linking vitamin D deficiency with hypertension and cardiovascular disease in general.

The first evidence suggesting a possible relationship between vitamin D and hypertension came from the INTERSALT study, which evaluated the relationship between blood pressure and electrolyte excretion in 10079 subjects from different countries [12].The study found a direct relationship between systolic and diastolic blood pressure and the distance from the equator, and hypothesized that the synthesis of vitamin D by ultraviolet light could play a role in these differences. This hypothesis was confirmed by a small study in 18 patients who were randomized to treatment with alpha or beta ultraviolet light. The group receiving beta ultraviolet light showed a statistically-significant reduction in systolic and diastolic blood pressure measured by ambulatory blood-pressure monitoring (ABPM) associated with an increase of 162% in plasma 25-vitamin D [13].

Numerous subsequent studies have tried to demonstrate an association between vitamin D and hypertension. Initial studies had a small sample size and inconsistent results. Some showed an inverse relationship, some neutral results and some a direct relationship. However, these studies could be criticized methodologically, mainly due to the small number of patients included [14].

Since 2007, some cohort studies, which provide more valid data, have been carried out.

Three studies have examined the relationship between vitamin D and hypertension using data from the NHAMES III (Third National Health and Nutrition Examination Survey). Scragg et al [15] studied 12644 people aged ≥ 20 years not on antihypertensive treatment. Patients were divided into quintiles of vitamin D levels, with those in the highest quintile presenting lower blood pressure levels, (-3 mmHg systolic blood pressure and -1.6 mmHg diastolic blood pressure). The effect was greater in people aged > 50 years. Judd et al [16] analyzed 7699 NHAMES III subjects and stratified them into five categories according to the Joint National Committee 7 recommendations (normal blood pressure <120 mmHg, prehypertension 120-129 mmHg, prehypertension, borderline, 130-139 mmHg, stage I hypertension 140-159 mmHg, stage II hypertension> 160 mmHg). They measured vitamin D levels in all patients at different times of the year and found a statistically-significant association between circulating vitamin D levels and systolic hypertension. The significance disappeared when age and the black population were analysed. Causcasian patients with levels of 25-vitamin D > 80 nmol/l had a 20%-lower systolic blood pressure than patients with vitamin D < 50 nmol/l. Martins et al [17], studied 15088 (7816 men and 7902 women) NHAMES subjects to determine the relationship between vitamin D and vascular risk factors, including hypertension. They found lower levels of vitamin D in patients with a history of hypertension (30 ng/ml vs 28 ng/ml, p = 0.001). Dividing the study subjects by quartiles of vitamin D levels showed that subjects in the first quartile (vitamin D <21 ng/ml) had a 30%-higher risk of hypertension than subjects in the fourth quartile (vitamin D> 37 ng/ml), OR 1.31 (95% CI 1.13-1.41, p = 0.01). Recently, Zhao et al [18], using the same database, analyzed the role of vitamin D and PTH (parathormone) in a cross-sectional study of 5414 subjects after excluding patients receiving antihypertensive therapy. Serum vitamin D levels were significantly lower and PTH levels higher in patients with hypertension and prehypertension. The regression model showed that the association remained statistically-significant for vitamin D after accounting for PTH, and that PTH remained significant after accounting for vitamin D. This suggests that 25-vitamin D and PTH are independently associated with prehypertension and hypertension.

Another American study analyzed the relationship between vitamin D and hypertension in 117730 subjects from the Health Professionals Follow-up Study and the Nurse's Health Study [19] using both cross-sectional and longitudinal analyses. The cross-sectional analysis found an inverse relationship between blood pressure and vitamin D. The longitudinal analysis established two cut-off points (25-vitamin D < 15 ng/ml and < 30 ng/ml) and found that subjects with levels <15 had a 3-fold risk of developing hypertension (6-fold in males and 2.5-fold in females). The main limitation of the longitudinal study was that vitamin D levels were measured in a limited number of subjects and the results extrapolated to the whole study population.

These results were reproduced in European studies. A German cohort study of 1763 males and 2267 females found lower levels of 25-OH vitamin D in women with hypertension [20]. Hyppönen et al [21] studied the relationship between vitamin D, metabolic syndrome and its components, including hypertension, in a UK cohort aged > 45 years. Subjects were divided into tertiles based on levels of vitamin D, and the results showed a reduced risk of hypertension in the highest tertile (OR 0.72, 95% CI 0.61-0.86). The LASA (Longitudinal Aging Study Amsterdam) cohort study, which included 1205 subjects aged > 65 years found no relationship between levels of 25-OH vitamin D and blood pressure. However, participants had high levels of vitamin D, which may explain the lack of relationship [22].

The Tromso (Norway) cohort study conducted a transversal and longitudinal analyses in 4125 subjects. The transversal study found an inverse relationship between vitamin D levels and systolic blood pressure. However, unlike the similar American study [19], the longitudinal arm did not find that low vitamin D levels were predictive of the development of hypertension, although the methodology was different [23].

The Australian Geelong cohort study of 861 women aged 20- 92 years found similar results [24]. Women in the lowest tertile of vitamin D levels had higher blood pressure. A Chinese study found no association between vitamin D and hypertension, but did find an association with PTH. They studied 939 men aged < 65 years with high vitamin D levels, which may explain the negative results found [25].

A recent meta-analysis examined the relationship between 25-OH vitamin D and hypertension and included 18 studies (3 prospective case-control, one prospective cohort and 14 cross-sectional) contained in 15 articles. Fourteen studies showed an inverse association between 25-OH vitamin D and hypertension, with 10 studies showing a statistically-significant association and four showing a non-significant direct association. Multivariate analysis adjusted between categories of vitamin D (high versus low) found that the OR of hypertension for patients with higher levels of vitamin D was 0.73 (95% CI 0.63 to 0.84), although the results of the various studies were heterogeneous. The relationship remained after adjustment for ethnicity, but only studies in Caucasians showed no heterogeneity. A dose-response analysis found that, for an increase in vitamin D of more than 40 nmol/l, the OR for hypertension was 0.78 (95% CI 0.67 to 0.92) but with wide heterogeneity between studies, except those conducted in Caucasians. The results confirmed the inverse relationship between serum levels of vitamin D and hypertension [26].

The data from the cohort studies show an association between vitamin D levels and blood pressure levels. Hypertensive patients have lower vitamin D levels and blood pressure was lower in patients with higher levels of vitamin D.

Vitamin D and Hypertension: Biological Mechanisms

Two methods can be used to try to prove the causality of the association between vitamin D and hypertension: biological plausibility (pathophysiological mechanisms which may explain the association), and the therapeutic response to vitamin D supplementation in methodologically-sound studies.

Various biological mechanisms have been implicated in this association: activation of the renin-angiotensin-aldosterone system (RAAS), endothelial dysfunction, secondary hyperparathyroidism and insulin resistance.

Activation of the renin-angiotensin-aldosterone system. The RAAS plays a key role in regulating blood pressure, and its various components are therapeutic targets for the treatment of hypertension. RAAS activation causes reabsorption of sodium and water and peripheral arterial vasoconstriction, mechanisms which both increase blood pressure. Vitamin D receptors are distributed throughout the body, including the juxtaglomerular apparatus, the main site of renin synthesis. The active form of vitamin D, 1,25-dihydroxy-vitamin D, may increase cytosolic calcium levels in renal tubular cells and may therefore reduce renal renin secretion [27]. Li et al [28] found that vitamin D regulation of renin was independent of the calcium metabolism and that 1,25 vitamin D suppressed renin transcription by a VDR-mediated mechanism in cell cultures.

Evidence from clinical studies has demonstrated an inverse relationship between circulating vitamin D levels and plasma renin activity [29,30]. Recently, Forman et al [31] studied the relationship between 25-OH vitamin D and various RAAS components in 184 normotensive subjects. Patients were divided into three groups according to vitamin D levels, normal (> 30 ng/ml), insufficient (15-29 ng/ml) and deficient (<15 ng/ml). The two latter groups had higher levels of angiotensin II and a blunted response of renal plasma flow to angiotensin II infusion, findings consistent with RAAS activation.

Endothelial dysfunction. Various studies have shown a relationship between vitamin D deficiency and endothelial dysfunction, as measured by the reduction in brachial artery flow-mediated dilation (FMD), and have found that this can be improved by vitamin D supplementation. Firstly, *in vitro* studies have shown that vitamin D can cause an imbalance between inflammatory and proinflammatory cytokines, reducing the activity of NF-kB, increasing production of IL-10 and lowering levels of IL-6, I L-1, interferon γ and TNF alpha [32]. Vitamin D deficiency could cause a predominance of inflammatory cytokines, favouring endothelial injury and the development of atherosclerosis. In order to test this hypothesis in humans, Jablonski et al [33] conducted a study of 47 men and 28 women, with a mean age of 62 years, who were divided into three groups based on levels of vitamin D. Brachial artery flow-mediated dilation was lower in patients with vitamin D insufficiency and deficiency, while endothelium-independent dilation did not differ between groups. In vitamin D deficient subjects, the expression of 1-alpha-hydroxylase and the vitamin D receptor was lower and the expression of NF-kB in vascular endothelial cells was higher, compared with subjects with normal vitamin D levels. Inhibition of NF-kB improved flow-mediated dilation. This study shows the first evidence in humans of a possible association between vitamin D deficiency and vascular endothelial inflammation with reduced expression of the vitamin D receptor and 1-alpha-hydroxylase. Secondly, endothelial cells contain vitamin D receptors, whose stimulation inhibits cell proliferation [34].

Secondary hyperparathyroidism. Vitamin D deficiency results in reduced intestinal calcium absorption, requiring increased PTH levels to maintain calcium levels within normal limits.

Observational studies have shown an association between hypertension and both primary and secondary hyperparathyroidism [35]. In secondary hyperparathyroidism, the relationship between PTH and hypertension has been shown to be independent of levels of vitamin D [18].

However, the exact mechanisms that would explain this association are not clear. PTH, through its binding to the PTH receptor, activates long-lasting (L)-type calcium channels, favouring their entry into the cell, and producing simultaneously the mobilization of calcium from the sarcoplasmic reticulum and a reduction in the calcium output to the exterior. This results in an overload of calcium within the cells [36].

This mechanism results in the induction of oxidative stress and the release of proinflammatory cytokines, which increase vascular rigidity and resistance, and thereby promote atherosclerotic changes [37,38].

The continuous infusion of PTH in healthy volunteers results in the occurrence of hypercalcemia and hypertension [39]. If calcium is administered subsequently to lower levels of PTH, the blood pressure is normalized [40]. The possible involvement of the renin-angiotensin aldosterone system has been suggested.

Some studies [41,42] have shown that PTH increases plasma renin activity and the secretion of aldosterone and cortisol, all mechanisms which raise blood pressure, although other studies are not in agreement. Moreover, in hypertensive patients with primary hyperparathyroidism, parathyroidectomy results in a reduction in both systolic and diastolic blood pressure.

However, Bollerslev et al [43] found no differences in blood pressure levels and parameters of insulin resistance between patients who did or did not receive this type of surgery. Taken together, these results suggest a role for the influence of PTH on blood pressure.

Insulin resistance. The presence of vitamin D receptors in pancreatic beta cells suggests that these cells might act as regulators of insulin secretion. In in vitro studies and experimental models, it has been observed that vitamin D is essential in the release of insulin in response to glucose and the maintenance of glucose tolerance.

Epidemiological studies suggest an association between vitamin D levels and the risk of hyperglycemia and/or insulin resistance [44]. Chonchol et al [45] described an association between vitamin D deficiency, insulin resistance and an increased risk of diabetes. The Framingham cohort study found an inverse correlation between vitamin D deficiency, glucose and insulin levels after adjusting for several variables [46].

The mechanism of the association of low vitamin D levels and insulin resistance is not completely clear. One beneficial effect of vitamin D may be to stimulate the expression of insulin receptors and enhance the response of glucose transport to the interior of the cell. In addition, vitamin D regulates the intracellular and extracellular levels of calcium, which are essential to processes mediated by insulin in the adipose tissue and muscle.

Finally, vitamin D deficiency may induce an inflammatory response that increases insulin resistance [47]. PTH could increase insulin resistance and thereby constitute an additional mechanism that could increase blood pressure.

Figure 1 shows a representation of the factors discussed.

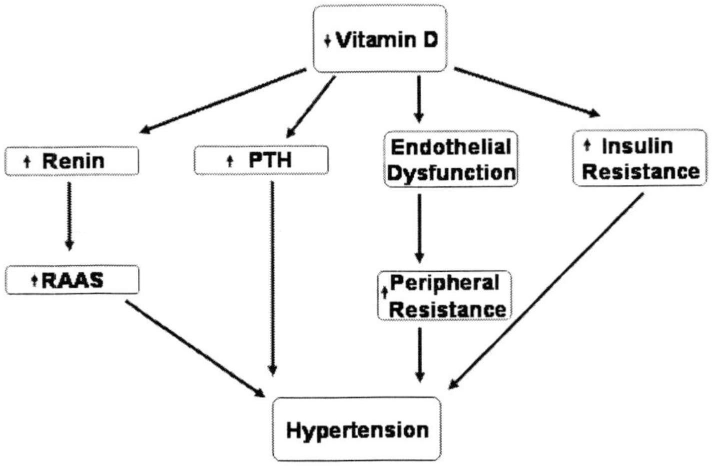

Figure 1. Relationship between hypertension and vitamin D: biological mechanisms.

Vitamin D and the Antihypertensive Response

The first study to examine the effect of vitamin D on hypertension was conducted in China. Pan et al [48] assessed the blood pressure response after administration of vitamin D supplements in 54 elderly, institutionalized patients aged > 65 years who were randomized to 4 groups (calcium, vitamin D, calcium and vitamin D, and placebo) The dose used was 200 IU/day with a follow-up period of 11 weeks. Vitamin D did not reduce blood pressure when compared with placebo. A subsequent English study [49] included 94 patients in the treatment group and 94 in the placebo group with a mean age of 70 years (range 63 to 76). The study was conducted in winter when vitamin D levels are lowest. The treatment group received 2.5 mg (100000 IU) of vitamin D in a single dose and were followed for 5 weeks. An increase in vitamin D levels and a decrease in PTH with no change in blood pressure were found in both groups.

Methodologically, the best study was that made by Pfeiffer et al [50], which included 148 subjects aged >70 years without hypertension and with vitamin D levels < 50 nmol/l. Patients were randomized to two groups, calcium (600 mg/day) and calcium (600 mg/day) with vitamin D (400 IU/day). The study was conducted in March, the month when vitamin D levels are lowest in Germany, and lasted for 8 weeks. Patients treated with vitamin D showed an increase in vitamin D, a reduction in PTH and a reduction in systolic blood pressure of 9.2% ($p = 0.02$). Systolic blood pressure fell by more than 5 mmHg in 81% of patients receiving vitamin D compared with 47% of those receiving only calcium. In an elderly population without known hypertension and deficient in vitamin D, calcium supplementation and vitamin D significantly reduced systolic blood pressure. This suggests a possible role of vitamin D in the pathogenesis of hypertension in this population.

In 2007, Major et al [51] published a study in obese women with a mean age of 43 years whose main objective was to assess the effect of calcium and vitamin D3 (600 mg calcium and 400 IU vitamin D) on weight and the lipid profile during a period of 15 weeks. The secondary objective was to evaluate the effects on blood pressure. The results showed a reduction in blood pressure in the active treatment group. One bias of this study was that treated patients lost more weight than the placebo group, and weight is known to affect blood pressure.

A recently-published study [52] with a very-small sample size of 7 subjects evaluated the effect of calcitriol (activated vitamin D) on blood pressure and found a reduction in systolic blood pressure of 9% in patients receiving calcitriol. The effect disappeared after withdrawal of calcitriol. There was no effect in the groups receiving placebo or inactivated vitamin D. The results are interesting but of little value due to the sample size and the follow-up period of only 3 weeks.

All the aforementioned studies have a small sample size, a short follow-up period and heterogeneous populations and therefore the results are mixed. To resolve these issues, the most useful option would be to design a study with a homogeneous population, large sample size and adequate follow-up. Another possibility would be to group these small studies and perform a meta-analysis.

The Women's Health Initiative [53] is a randomized, placebo-controlled study that evaluated the effect of calcium and vitamin D supplements over a long follow-up period on various aspects of women's health, including hypertension, in 36282 postmenopausal women. The active treatment group received 1000 mg/day of calcium and 400 IU of vitamin D3, although both the active and the placebo group were allowed to continue with previous nutritional supplements. Therefore, there were women in the placebo group who were taking calcium and vitamin D. During the 7 years of the study, no differences in either systolic blood pressure ($p = 0.14$) or diastolic blood pressure ($p = 0.20$) were found. Dividing the population into subgroups (age, race, education, previous blood pressure, physical activity, BMI, total calcium intake, total vitamin D intake, compliance) showed no differences. The development of hypertension during the study was similar in both groups. The study concluded that there was no effect of supplemental calcium and vitamin D on the occurrence or reduction of hypertension. Although the study was solid, it had some limitations. The placebo group included subjects who were already taking vitamin D supplements and the population included only postmenopausal women.

Two meta-analyses have tried to resolve the question of the possible benefits of vitamin D in reducing blood pressure. The first is a systematic review, which conducted a meta-analysis of studies that could be pooled quantitatively. The search strategy consisted of controlled, randomized studies which compared vitamin D and placebo, with reduced blood pressure being the main outcome. Active treatment was considered in addition to the different forms of vitamin D, including ultraviolet light. Eleven studies that met fulfilled the selection criteria and were all carried out in non-institutionalized individuals from western Europe were included, together with a single study of institutionalized patients conducted in Taiwan. Of the eleven studies from western Europe, the meta-analysis finally included only eight studies in which mean baseline blood pressure was > 140 mmHg [54]. It included 545 patients and found that vitamin D supplementation resulted in a small, non-significant reduction in systolic blood pressure (-3.6 mmHg, 95% CI -0.8 to 0.7, $p = 0.1$), although there was wide heterogeneity between studies. There was also a small, statistically-significant reduction in diastolic blood pressure (-3.1 mmHg, 95% CI -5.5 to -0.6), $p = 0.01$) although heterogeneity persisted. These data would invalidate the meta-analysis.

Three studies did not present raised blood pressure levels at baseline, and showed no benefits for vitamin D supplements. A subgroup analysis compared the effectiveness of inactivated forms of vitamin D (vitamin D2, vitamin D3 and ultraviolet light) versus active forms (calcitriol/1-alpha-calcidiol). The inactivated forms were associated with a statistically significant reduction in blood pressure (-6.2 mmHg, 95% CI -12.32-0.04, p = 0.05), while the active forms of vitamin D showed no effect. Neither of the two forms (activated and inactivated) had an effect on diastolic blood pressure. The meta-analysis showed a reduction in diastolic blood pressure in hypertensive patients taking vitamin D supplements and the reduction was greatest in patients taking the inactivated forms of vitamin D, where there was also a reduction in systolic blood pressure.

Another recently published meta-analysis included 4 studies using vitamin D3 supplements [55]. Fewer patients (429) were included, with a follow-up of 5-15 weeks, but with no heterogeneity between studies. The results showed a reduction in systolic blood pressure of 2.44 mmHg (95% CI -4.86 to -0.02) but no reduction in diastolic blood pressure.

The published data are inconclusive and do not confirm or disprove the potential benefits of vitamin D on BP. The studies are small, with different populations, different doses of vitamin D and short follow-up periods. This means that all meta-analyses so far are of poor quality. The only methodologically-robust study with a large sample size found no benefit at a dose of 400 IU/day, although the population was limited to postmenopausal women and the placebo group was biased. Higher quality studies, with higher doses of vitamin D (800 IU/day) targeting older populations deficient in vitamin D are required before conclusions can be drawn regarding this important question.

References

[1] Holick MF. Sunlight and vitamin D for bone health and prevention of autoinmune diseases, cancer and cardiovascular disease. *Am. J. Clin. Nutr.* 2004; 80:1678-88.

[2] Zittermann A. Vitamin D and disease prevention with special reference to cardiovascular disease. *Prog. Biophys. Mol. Biol.* 2006; 92:39-48.

[3] Kato S, Kim MS, Yamakoaka K, Fujiki R. Mechanisms of transcriptional repression by 1,25(OH)2 vitamin D. *Curr. Opin. Nephrol. Hypertens.* 2007 Jul;16:297-304.

[4] Fahrleitner A, Dobnog H, Obermosterer A, et al. Vitamin D deficiency and secondary hyperparathyroidism are common complications in patients with peripheral arterial disease. *J. Gen. Intern. Med.* 2002; 17: 633-639.

[5] Pérez-Castrillón JL, Vega G, Abad L et al. The effects of atorvastatin on vitamin D levels in patients with acute ischemic heart disease. *Am. J. Cardiol.* 2007; 99:903-905.

[6] Pérez Castrillón JL, Gómez Alonso C. Métodos de determinación de la vitamina D y valores de normalidad. *REEMO* 2005; 14: 19-23.

[7] Rosen CL. Vitamin D insufficiency. *N. Engl. J. Med.* 2011; 364: 248-254.

[8] Guinde AA, Liu MC, Camargo CA. Demographic differences and trends of vitamin D insufficiency in the US population, 1988-2004. *Arch. Intern. Med.* 2009; 169: 626-632.

[9] Niño V, Perez Castrillón JL. Niveles de vitamina D en población mayor de 65 años. *REEMO* 2008; 17:1-4.

[10] Quesada JM, Sans I, Benito P, Jimenez JA, Bouillon R. Vitamin D status of elderly people in Spain. *Age Ageing* 1989; 18: 392-397.

[11] Gomez Alonso C, Naves Diez ML, Fernandez Martin JL, Diaz Lopez JB, Fernandez M, Cannata Andia J. Vitamin D status and secondary hyperparathyroidism. The importance of 25-hydroxivitamin D cut-off levels. *Kidney Int.* 2003; 85: 44-48.

[12] Intersalt Cooperative Research Group, Intersalt: an international study of electrolyte excretion and blood pressure. Results for 24 hour urinary sodium and potassium excretion. *BMJ* 297: 319-328, 1998.

[13] Krause R, Bürhing M, Hopfenmüller W, Holick MF, Dharma AM. Ultraviolet B and blood pressure. *Lancet* 1998; 352: 709-710.

[14] Iftekhar M, Uwaifo GI, Nicholas WC, Koch CA. Does vitamin D deficiency cause hypertension? Current evidence from clinical studies and potential mechanisms. *International Journal of Endocrinology*, 2010 ID 579640.

[15] Scragg R, Sowers M, Bell C. Serum 25-hydroxyvitamin D, ethnicity and blood pressure in the third National Health and Nutrition Examination Survey. *Am. J. Hypertens* 2007; 20: 713-719.

[16] Judd SE, Nanes MS, Ziegler TR, Wilson PW, Tangpricha V. Optimal vitamin D status attenuates the age-associated increase in systolic blood pressure in white Americans: results from the third National Health and Nutrition Examination Survey. *Am. J. Clin. Nutr.* 2008; 87: 136-141.

[17] Martins D, Wolf M, Pen D, et al. Prevalence of cardiovascular risk factors and the serum levels of 25-hydroxyvitamin D in the United States: data from the third National Health and Nutrition Examination Survey. *Arch. Intern. Med.* 2007; 167: 1159-1165.

[18] Zhao G, Ford ES, Li C, Kris-Etherton PM, Etherton TD, Balluz LS. Independent associations of serum concentrations of 25-hydroxyvitamin D and parathyroid hormone with blood pressure among US adults. *J. Hypertens* 2010; 28: 1821-1828.

[19] Forman JP, Giovannucci E, Holmes MD, Bischoff-Ferrari HA, Tworoger SS, Willett WC, Curhan GC. Plasma 25-hydroxyvitamin D levels and risk of incident hypertension. *Hypertension* 2007; 49: 1063-1069.

[20] Hintzpeter B, Mensink GB, Thierfelder W, Müller MJ, Scheidt-Nave C. Vitamin D status and health correlates among German adults. *Eur. J. Clin. Nutr.* 2008; 62: 1079-1089.

[21] Hyppönen E, Boucher BJ, Berry DJ, Power C. 25-hydroxyvitamin D, IGF-1 and metabolic syndrome at 45 years of age: a cross-sectional study in the 1958 British Birth Cohort. *Diabetes* 2008; 57: 298-305.

[22] Snijder MB, Lips P, Seidell JC, Visser M, Deeg DGH, DeDekker JM, Van Dam RM. Vitamin D status and parathyroid hormone levels in relation to blood pressure: a population-based study in older men and women. *J. Intern. Med.* 2007; 261: 558-565.

[23] Jorde R, Figenschau Y, Emaus N, Hutchinson M, Grimnes G. Serum 25-hydroxyvitamin D levels are strongly related to systolic blood pressure but do not predict future hypertension. *Hypertension* 2010; 55: 792-798.

[24] Pasco JA, Henry MJ, Nicholson GC, Brennan SL, Kotowicz MA. Behavioural and physical characteristics associated with vitamin D status in women. *Bone* 2009; 44: 1085-1091.

[25] Chan R, Dan D, Woo J et al. Serum 25-hydroxyvitamin D and parathyroid hormone levels in relation to blood pressure in a cross-sectional study in older Chinese men. *J. Hum. Hypertens* 2011; doi:10.1038/jhh.2010.126.

[26] Burgaz A, Orsini N, Larsson SC, Wolk A. Blood 25-hydroxyvitamin D concentration and hypertension: a meta-analysis *J. Hypertens* 2011; doi: 10.1097/HJHob013e 3283432019.

[27] Li YC, Qiao G, Uskokovic M,Xiang W, Zheng W, Kong J. Vitamin D: a negative endocrine regulator of the renin-angiotensin system and blood pressure. *J. Steroid Biochem. Mol. Biol.* 2004; 89-90: 387-392.

[28] Li YC, Kong J, Wei M, Chen ZF, Liu SQ, Cao LP. 1,25-Dihydroxyvitamin D (3) is a negative endocrine regulator of the renin-angiotensin system. *J. Clin. Invest.* 2002; 110: 229-238.

[29] Resnick LM, Muller FB, Laragh JH. Calcium regulating hormones in essential hypertension: relation to plasma renin activity and sodium metabolism. *Ann. Intern. Med.* 1986; 105: 649-654.

[30] Burgess ED, Hawkins RG, Wanatabe M. Interaction of 1,25-dihidroxyvitamin D and plasma renin activity in high renin essential hypertension. *Am. J. Hypertens* 1990; 3: 903-905.

[31] Forman JP, Williams JS, Fisher N. Plasma 25-hydroxyvitamin D and regulation of the rennin-angiotensin system in humans. *Hypertension* 2010; 55: 1283-1288.

[32] Zittermann A, Scheleithoff SS, Koerfer R. Vitamin D insufficiency in congestive heart failure: Why and what to do about it ? *Heart Fail Rev.* 2006; 11: 25-33.

[33] Jabolnski KL, Chonchol M, Pierce GL, Walker AE, Seals DR. 25-Hydroxyvitamin D deficiency is associated with inflammation-linked vascular endothelial dysfunction in middle-aged and older adults. *Hypertension* 2011; 57:63-69.

[34] Wong MS, Delansorne R, Man RY et al. Vitamin D derivatives acutely reduce endothelium-dependent contractions in the aorta of the spontaneously hypertensive rat. *Am. J. Physiol. Heart Circ. Physiol.* 2008; 295: H289-H296.

[35] Nainby-Luxmoore JC, Langford HG, Nelson NC, Watson RL, Barnes TY. A case-comparison study of hypertension and hyperparathyroidism. *J. Clin. Endocrinol. Metab.* 1982; 55: 303-306.

[36] Smogorzewski M, Zayed M, Zhang YB et al. Parathyroid hormone increases cytosolic calcium concentration in adult rat cardiac myocytes. *Am. J. Physiol.* 1993; 264:H1998-H2006.

[37] Rubin MR, Maurer MS, McMahon DJ, Bilezikian JP, Silverberg SJ. Arterial stiffness in mild primary hyperparathyroidism. *J. Clin. Endocrinol. Metab.* 2005; 90; 3326-3320.

[38] Fitzpatrick LA, Bilezikian JP, Silverberg SJ. Parathyroid hormone and the cardiovascular system. *Curr. Osteoporos Rep.* 2008; 6: 77-83.

[39] Hulter HN, Melby JC, Peterson JC, Cooke CR. Chronic continuous PTH infusion results in hypertension in normal patients. *J. Clin. Hypertens* 1986; 2:360-370.

[40] Kamycheva E, Jorde R, Haug E, Sager G, Sundsfjord J. Effects of acute hypercalcemia on blood pressure in patients with and without parathyroid secretion. *Acta Physiol. Scand.* 2005; 184: 113-119.

[41] Kovacs L, Goth MI, Szabolcs I, Dohan O, Ferencz A, Szilagy G. The effect of surgical treatment on secondary hyperaldosteronism and relative hyperinsulinemia in primary hyperparathyroidism. *Eur. J. Endocrinol.* 1998; 138:543-7.

[42] Gennari C, Nami R, Gonnelli S. Hypertension and primary hyperparathyroidism: the role of adrenergic and rennin-angiotensin-aldosterone systems. *Miner Electrolyte Metab.* 1995; 21: 77-81.

[43] Bollerslev J, Jansson S, Mollerup CL, et al. Medical observation, compared with parathyroidectomy, for asymptomatic primary hyperparathyroidism: a prospective, randomized trial. *J. Clin. Endocrinol. Metab.* 2007; 92: 1687-1692.

[44] Alvarez JA, Ashraf AP, Hunter GR, Gower BA. Serum 25-hydroxyvitamin D and parathyroid hormone are independent determinants of whole-body insulin sensitivity in women and may contribute to lower insulin sensitivity in African Americans. *Am. J. Clin. Nutr.* 2010; 92: 1344-1349.

[45] Chonchol M, Scragg R. 25-hydroxyvitamin D, insulin, resistance and kidney function in the Third National Health and Nutrition Examination Survey. *Kidney International* 2007; 71: 134-139.

[46] Liu E, Meigs JB, Pittas AG, McKeown NM, Economos CD, Booth SL, Jacques PF. Plasma 25-hydroxivitamin D is associated with markers of the insulin resistant phenotype in nondiabetic adults. *J. Nutr.* 2009; 139: 329-334.

[47] Shoelson SE, Herrero L, Naaz A. Obesity, inflammation and insulin resistance. *Gastroenterology* 2007; 132: 2017-2019.

[48] Pan WH, Wang CY, Li LA et al. No significant effect of calcium and vitamin D supplementation on blood pressure and calcium metabolism in elderly Chinese. *Chin. J. Physiol.* 1993; 36: 85-94.

[49] Scragg R, Khaw KT, Murphy S. Effect of winter oral vitamin D3 supplementation on cardiovascular risk factors in elderly adults. *Eur. J. Clin. Nutr.* 1995; 49: 640-646.

[50] Pfeifer M, Begerow B, Minne HW et al. Effects of a short-term vitamin D (3) and calcium supplementation on blood pressure and parathyroid hormone levels in elderly women. *J. Clin. Endocrinol. Metab.* 2001; 86: 1633-1637.

[51] Major GC, Alarie F, Doré J et al. Supplementation with calcium + vitamin D enhances the beneficial effect of weight loss on plasma lipid and lipoprotein concentrations. *Am. J. Clin. Nutr.* 2007; 85: 54-59.

[52] Judd SE, Raiser SN, Kumari M, Tangpricha V. 1,25-dihydroxyvitamin D3 reduces systolic blood pressure in hypertensive adult: a pilot feasibility study. *J. Est. Biochem. Mol. Biol.* 2010; 121: 445-447.

[53] Margolis KL, Ray RM, Van Horn L et al. Effect of calcium and vitamin supplementation on blood pressure: The Women's Health Initiative Randomized Trial. *Hypertension* 2008; 32: 847-855.

[54] Witham MD, Nadir MA, Struthers AD. Effect of vitamin D on blood pressure: a systematic review and meta-analysis. *J. Hypertens* 2009: 27:1948-1954.

[55] Hui Wu S, Co SC, Zhong L. Effects of vitamin D supplementation on blood pressure. *South Med. J.* 2010; 103: 729-737.

In: Vitamin D Deficiency
Editors: V. Lerner and C. Miodownik

ISBN: 978-1-61470-964-0

Chapter IV

Vitamin D Deficiency and Cardiovascular Disease

***Arie Steinvil*[*,1,2], *Itzhak Shapira*[1,2] *and Ori Rogowski*[1,2]**

[1]Departments of Internal Medicine "D" and "E", Tel-Aviv Sourasky Medical Center, Israel

[2]Sackler Faculty of Medicine, Tel-Aviv University, Tel-Aviv, Israel

Abstract

Accumulating data over the past few years suggest that vitamin D deficiency has an adverse effect on cardiovascular health and that the prevalence of vitamin D deficiency is significantly higher among patients with cardiovascular disease (CVD) risk factors, contributing to the pathogenesis of CVD. Vitamin D has pluripotent cardiovascular effects. The activity of its receptors has been associated with blood pressure regulation through inhibition of vascular smooth muscle proliferation, down-regulation of myocyte proliferation and their hypertrophy, cardiac muscle contractility, decrease in plasma renin activity, anti-inflammatory properties, as well as cholesterol synthesis and hydroxylation. There is no convincing proof that vitamin D supplementation with the intent to lower the number of cardiovascular events is beneficial. Thus, despite the promise of vitamin D in disease prevention, as suggested by a number of studies, the evidence for widespread use of high-dose vitamin D supplementation in the general population remains insufficient. The cardiovascular risk associated with vitamin D deficiency has been demonstrated regardless of the amount of exposure to the sun, suggesting the possibility that vitamin D deficiency could be a biomarker of a lifestyle that lacks outdoor activities rather than the cause of increased CVD risk.

[*] Correspondence author: Arie Steinvil, MD, MHA. Department of Internal Medicine "D", Tel-Aviv Sourasky Medical Center, affiliated to the Sackler Faculty of Medicine, Tel-Aviv University, Tel-Aviv, Israel. Mailing address: 6 Weizmann Street, Tel-Aviv, 64239 Israel. Tel.: +972 3 6973313; Fax: +972 3 6973885; Email: arikst@tasmc.health.gov.il.

Keywords: Vitamin D; Vitamin D deficiency; Cardiovascular disease; Cardiovascular mortality

Abbreviations

CVD	cardiovascular disease;
VDR	vitamin D receptor;
PTH	parathyroid hormone;
UV	ultraviolet;
IHD	ischemic heart disease;
NHANES	national health and nutrition examination survey;
HDL	high-density lipoproteins;
LDL	high-density lipoproteins;
HR	hazard ratio;
RR	relative risk

Introduction

Mounting evidence has been accumulating on the association between vitamin D deficiency and cardiovascular disease (CVD) risk factors and CVD morbidity [1-7]. The actual role of vitamin D in CVD and its risk factors, however, is still unknown. Lower levels of vitamin D have been associated with a higher prevalence of acute myocardial infarction [6, 8], acute stroke [9, 10], congestive heart failure [11], peripheral vascular disease [12, 13], diabetes mellitus [14] and hypertension [15]. A meta-analysis of 18 randomized controlled trials comprising 57,000 individuals showed that vitamin D intake marginally improved all-cause mortality, partly by decreasing CVD deaths [16]. Wang et al have shown a similar benefit in five prospective studies of patients receiving dialysis and in one study involving the general population [17]. A recent meta-analysis of 28 studies that included 99,745 participants found that the highest levels of vitamin D were associated with a 43% reduction in cardio-metabolic disorders[18].

High levels of vitamin D among middle-age and elderly populations were reported to be associated with a substantial decrease in CVD, type 2 diabetes and metabolic syndrome [18]. Vitamin D supplementation did not, however, reduce CVD events or mortality in the women's health initiative trial of 36,282 female participants [19]. Similarly, a recent meta-analysis conducted to examine the association between vitamin D status, including the effect of vitamin D supplementation, and cardio-metabolic outcomes in generally healthy adults showed no clinically significant effect of vitamin D supplementation at the dosages given [20].

Thus, current recommended levels of serum 25(OH)D, which are primarily based on levels needed to maintain optimum bone health and prevent rickets [21], might not be associated with the levels of vitamin D that may be necessary to minimize the prevalence of CVD and its risk factors. These discouraging findings serve to even further intensify the debate on the need of vitamin D supplementation for CVD prevention or on the role of vitamin D as a cardiac biomarker [22].

Vitamin D has a pluripotent effect, with its receptors having been shown to be present in many tissues in the body, including the heart and vascular bed [2]. The activity of these receptors has been associated with blood pressure regulation through inhibition of vascular smooth muscle proliferation, down-regulation of myocyte proliferation and their hypertrophy [23], regulation of plasma renin activity [24], as well as anti-inflammatory properties [25]. Furthermore, variants in proximity to genes involved in cholesterol synthesis might identify individuals with increased risk of vitamin D insufficiency [26].

Although reduced sun exposure has been related to vitamin D deficiency, cardiovascular risk associated with vitamin D deficiency has been demonstrated regardless of the amount of solar exposure in a western society [27]. Thus vitamin D deficiency might reflect lack of sun exposure due to a principally indoor lifestyle that, in combination with a lack of physical activity, leads to an increased risk for the development of obesity, metabolic syndrome and CVD risk factors. Therefore, the possibility exists that vitamin D deficiency could be a biomarker of a passive lifestyle rather than the cause of increased CVD risk [1].

Vitamin D Role in Cardiovascular Pathophysiology

The role of vitamin D in regulating calcium and phosphate metabolism in the intestine, kidney, and bone has been known for several decades. Over the last decade, studies have provided evidence that vitamin D may also play an important role in regulating metabolism in other organs, including the heart and blood vessels [28]. This role has been suggested by the identification of a specific receptor (the vitamin D receptor, VDR) for 1,25-dihydroxyvitamin D, the active metabolite of vitamin D, in these tissues [29], as well as by the presence of a vitamin D-dependent calcium-binding protein [30-32]. 1,25-dihydroxyvitamin D controls more than 200 genes, including genes responsible for the regulation of cellular proliferation, differentiation, apoptosis, and angiogenesis [30-32].

Effects on contractility and myocardium. Vitamin D-dependent calcium-binding protein is present on cardiac muscle and endothelial and vascular smooth muscle cells [1]. Vitamin D appears to be involved in calcium-dependent cellular processes, including the synthesis of calcium-binding protein, the activation of adenylate cyclase, the rapid activation of voltage-dependent calcium channels, and the influx, reuptake, and release of calcium from the sarcoplasmic reticulum [33]. Weishaar and Simpson [34] have shown that the changes in in-vitro cardiac contractile function that accompany vitamin D deficiency could not be prevented by preventing the hypocalcemia that normally accompanies vitamin D depletion, nor could they be reversed by restoration of serum calcium to normal levels after the initial period of vitamin D depletion in rats. In contrast, the change in in-vitro vascular muscle contractile function observed in vitamin D-deficient hypocalcemic rats could be prevented by maintaining serum calcium at normal levels and also reversed by restoration of serum calcium to normal after an initial period of vitamin D deficiency. These observations indicate that hypocalcemia does not account for the changes in cardiac contractile function that result from vitamin D depletion, and suggest a direct role for vitamin D in regulating cardiac contractility.

O'Connell et al have shown that vitamin D inhibits myocyte maturation, regulates myocyte proliferation and hypertrophy, in primary cultures of neonatal rat cardiomyocytes [23, 35]. Vitamin D increased myocyte protein levels and increased cell size, suggesting that it induces cardiac myocyte hypertrophy. The probable mechanism by which vitamin D regulates myocyte proliferation involves blocking entry into the S phase of the cell cycle. Induction of myocyte hypertrophy either in-vitro or in-vivo leads to an increase in VDR mRNA and protein levels [36]. Collectively, these findings suggest that the key components required for a functional vitamin D-dependent signaling system are present in the heart, and that this putatively anti-hypertrophic system is amplified in the setting of cardiac hypertrophy [36]. Xiang et al have shown that the size of left ventricular cardiomyocytes in VDR knockout (KO) mice was markedly increased compared with wild-type (WT) mice in parallel to the increase in the cardiac renin mRNA level, and amplified even further by angiotensin-converting enzyme inhibition, suggesting that both the systemic and cardiac renin-angiotensin systems support the notion that 1,25-dihydroxyvitamin D regulates cardiac functions [37].

Effects on vasculature. Vascular smooth muscle cells possess the enzyme 25(OH)D-1-hydroxylase, which also is up-regulated by parathyroid hormone (PTH) and estrogenic compounds, and are responsible for the conversion of vitamin D precursors into calcitriol [38, 39]. The expression of VDR in cultured bovine aortic endothelial and in venular and capillary endothelial cells of human skin biopsies has been documented as well [40]. Therefore, the presence of a vitamin D micro-endocrine system in endothelial cells, which consists of the coordinately regulated VDR and a 1 alpha-hydroxylase enzyme capable of producing 1,25(OH)D, suggests the existence of a vitamin D autocrine loop in endothelium and that it may play a role in the development or functions of this pathophysiologically significant cell population [40]. Vitamin D inhibits proliferation of vascular smooth muscle cells by an acute influx of Ca into the cells [41].

Watson et al have shown that vitamin D levels were inversely correlated with the extent of vascular calcification in 173 subjects at high and moderate risk for coronary heart disease [42]. After measuring aortic stiffness, brachial artery dispensability, and arterial calcification scores, London et al suggested that vitamin D deficiency could be associated with arteriosclerosis and endothelial dysfunction in patients who have end-stage renal disease and are on hemodialysis [43]. Vitamin D deficiency was associated with vascular calcifications and aortic stiffness in chronic and end stage renal disease [43-46], while, on the other hand, it increased matrix-γcarboxyglutamic acid protein (matrix Gla protein), a protein that protects against arterial calcification [47]. Vitamin D has also been found to suppress the synthesis and secretion of atrial natriuretic peptide [48, 49]. This inverse relation has been clearly demonstrated in heart failure patients [11]. Wang et al [26] showed that variants in close proximity to genes involved in cholesterol synthesis, hydroxylation and vitamin D transport affect the vitamin D status and help identify individuals at increased risk of vitamin D insufficiency. The novel gene locus DHCR7/ NADSYN1, which regulates cholesterol metabolism in the first step of synthesis, was found to be significantly associated with vitamin D levels [26].

Effects on Inflammation. Vitamin D exhibits systemic anti-inflammatory and immunomodulatory effects [50], as well as specific immunomodulatory ones on coronary vasculature [51]. One prospective cohort study demonstrated that low vitamin D levels were significantly correlated with C-reactive protein, interleukin 6, oxidative burden (serum phospholipid and glutathione), and cell adhesion (vascular cell adhesion molecule 1 and intercellular adhesion molecule 1) levels [52]. TNF-α-induced expression of intercellular adhesion molecule-1 and vascular cell adhesion molecule-1 in human endothelial cells are reportedly inhibited by vitamin D [53, 54]. Inflammatory processes were shown to play an important role in the development of adverse vascular events. Interleukin-6 and tumor necrosis factor physiological stimulants of C-reactive protein were suppressed by vitamin D [55], whereas the anti-inflammatory interleukin-10 was unregulated [25]. Suzuki et al examined the mRNA and protein expression of the vitamin D receptor in human coronary arterial endothelial cells by RT-PCR and Western blotting, respectively. Vitamin D significantly inhibited the TNF-α expression and NF-B in human coronary arterial endothelial cells, suggesting its role as a coronary artery inflammation modulator [51]. Inoue et al [56] and Wakasugi et al [57] had previously shown that vitamin D stimulates the production of prostacyclin by vascular smooth muscle cells, thus possibly preventing thrombus formation, cell adhesion, and smooth muscle cell proliferation.

Effect on Parathyroid hormone. A proposed mechanism by which lower vitamin D levels effect cardiovascular pathophysiology and prevalence of CVD is by secondary hyperparathyroidism. PTH, not unlike vitamin D, has been shown to have independent physiological cardiovascular effects and has been associated with CVD morbidity and mortality. PTH targets both cardiomyocytes and smooth muscle cells[58]. It activates protein kinase C (PKC) of cardiomyocytes via a PKC-activating domain previously identified on chondrocytes. Activation of PKC leads to hypertrophic growth and re-expression of fetal-type proteins in cardiomyocytes. PTH is an independent predictor of left ventricular hypertrophy [59]. It has also been linked to signal transduction, cardiomyocyte energy production and calcium influx [2]. PTH enzymatically up-regulates vitamin D in human vascular smooth muscle cells [38].

Multiple trials have demonstrated an independent association between elevated PTH due to primary or secondary causes and CVD. Hagstrom et al [60] demonstrated that plasma PTH levels predicted cardiovascular mortality in a study they conducted on a community-based cohort of elderly men (mean age, 71 years; n = 958) who were followed for a median of 9.7 years. In the same study, PTH predicted heart failure-associated hospitalizations, also after accounting for established risk factors and mineral metabolism variables and even in the absence of overt hyperparathyroidism [61]. Pilz et al [62] showed that PTH was associated with increased mortality and fatal cardiovascular events in patients referred for coronary angiography in the Ludwigshafen Risk and Cardiovascular Health Study on 3232 Caucasian patients followed for 7.7 years. Cawthon et al [63] reported that, in contrast to previous studies, lower vitamin D levels were not associated with an increased risk of all-cause or cause-specific mortality in older men, but that higher PTH levels were associated with a modest increase in mortality risk.

Vitamin D Deficiency and Cardiovascular Epidemiology

There are multiple lines of evidence to support a hypothetical association between low levels of vitamin D and a higher prevalence of CVD risk factors, morbidity and mortality. This association has been demonstrated by both direct and indirect means, i.e., indirectly by showing the association between lack of exposure to ultraviolet (UVB) light and between CVD, and directly in large cross-sectional and prospective studies.

Geography and CVD. The prevalence of CVD is affected by latitude, altitude and seasonally, all of which, in turn, affect individual exposure to ultraviolet light and indirectly to vitamin D levels. Thus, it is theoretically possible that there is an indirect link between the prevalence of CVD and vitamin D deficiency. Epidemiological studies reported that the rates of ischemic heart disease (IHD), cerebrovascular accidents, diabetes, hypertension as well as CVD death increase in proportion to increasing distance from the equator, as do those of vitamin D deficiency [47, 64] (Figures 1 and 2). Fleck described an increase in IHD with the increase in geographic latitude between death rates from IHD and geographic latitude in males and females from different European countries as well as from other Western countries [65]. Rich et al, however, found no difference in risk of major CVD between regions in the United States and no consistent association between myocardial infarction and CVD death and different regions [66]. A significantly increased risk of total stroke was, however, associated with residence in the southeastern United States compared with the northeast [66]. Generally, data on geographic latitude data are in agreement with the observation that environmental UVB radiation is absent from November until February at latitude 408N and from October until March at latitude 508N or 608N, while there is environmental UVB radiation throughout the year at latitude 308N or closer to the equator [67]. Winter values of serum vitamin D are higher in healthy subjects who live at lower latitudes compared with subjects living at higher ones [47].

UVB intensity increases exponentially with altitude [68]. Mortimer et al have shown a serial decline in mortality from IHD for males residing in the State of New Mexico, which is located at a relatively higher altitude [69]. An increase in altitude of 1000 meters (3280 feet) was associated with a 28% decrease in IHD mortality rates. Moreover, a statistical evaluation of different areas of the United States revealed an inverse association in death rates from IHD with altitude for both males and females [70]. Low mortality rates of IHD have also been reported for subjects living in Alpine European regions of high altitude [71].

Seasonality might also affect the prevalence of vitamin D deficiency as well as that of cardiovascular events. In Scotland, death rates of IHD in the summer were approximately 30% lower compared with those of the winter [72]. An evaluation of all IHD deaths in Scotland occurring between 1962 and 1971 also showed a winter peak and a summer nadir in male and female IHD deaths [72]. Data from the 1992 National British Household Survey found an inverse correlation between sunshine per year and IHD-caused death rate for males [73]. A United States survey examined the seasonal distributions of acute myocardial infarction in a regionally defined population (n = 103,322) monitored from 1980 to 1988: myocardial infarction occurred more frequently during the winter months from January to March compared with other months [74]. The reported data are compatible with results on the vitamin D status of healthy subjects living at geographic latitudes between 408N and 608N, e.g., in North America and Europe. These subjects had seasonal fluctuations in circulating vitamin D, with those in the summer being higher than those in the winter [47]. Seasonality of CVD has also been observed in the Southern hemisphere. One Australian study demonstrated that coronary events were 20–40% more likely to occur in the winter and spring than at other times of the year [75].

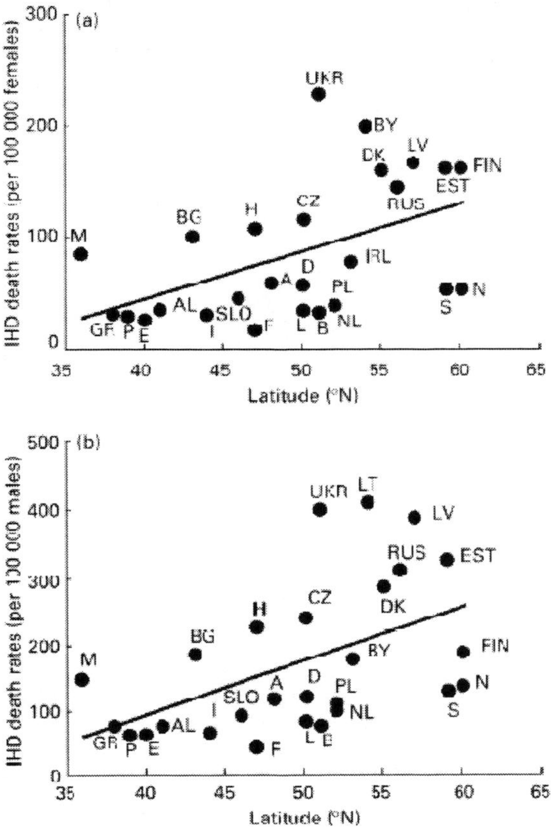

Figure 1. Associations between geographic latitude and IHD death rates in (a) females (r=0.49, P=0.01) and (b) males (r=51, P=0.01) of different European countries. A, Austria; AL, Albania; B, Belgium; BG, Bulgaria; BY, Belarus; CZ, Czech; D, Germany; DK, Denmark; E, Spain; EST, Estonia; F, France; FIN, Finland; GR, Greece; H, Hungary; I, Italy; L, Luxembourg; LT, Luthuania; LV, Latvia; M, Malta; N, Norway; NL, Netherlands; P, Portugal; PL, Poland; S, Sweden; SLO, Slovenia; RUS, Russia; UKR, Ukraine. Adopted with permission from Zittermann A," Putting cardiovascular disease and vitamin D insufficiency into perspective", British Journal of Nutrition 2005, volume 94(4), pages 483–492, Cambridge University press.

Similarly, Douglas et al have shown similar seasonal variation by month in coronary and cerebrovascular deaths in both sexes in a study comparing the southern hemisphere winter (June through August) with CVD morbidity nadir in the summer (December through February) [76]. Although climate change could explain the lack of sun exposure leading to vitamin D deficiency and perhaps cardiovascular morbidity, it has been previously demonstrated that seasonal CVD morbidity also fluctuates in populations living in sunny conditions year round. Kloner et al analyzed monthly death certificate data from Los Angeles County, California, for death caused by coronary artery disease between 1985 and 1996 (n = 222,265). Their results showed that there were seasonal variations in the development of coronary artery death even in the mild climate of Los Angeles County, with approximately 33% more deaths occurring in December and January than in June through September [77]. Similarly, Stienvil et al recently demonstrated that cardiovascular risk factors are prevalent in vitamin D deficiency in a population living in year-round sunny conditions[27]. Furthermore, since mean annual temperatures are lower in higher altitudes with concomitant relatively low

IHD mortality, temperature changes by themselves might not explain the seasonal variation in CVD morbidity [71]. Therefore, although cooler temperatures and sun exposure may play a role in vitamin D deficiency and prevalence of cardiovascular disease, other factors, such as winter infections [78] and their effect on inflammation [79, 80], a western lifestyle (which includes spending most of the daytime working hours in-door and infrequent sport activity, etc. could possibly explain association between a sunshine deficit to cardiovascular disease.

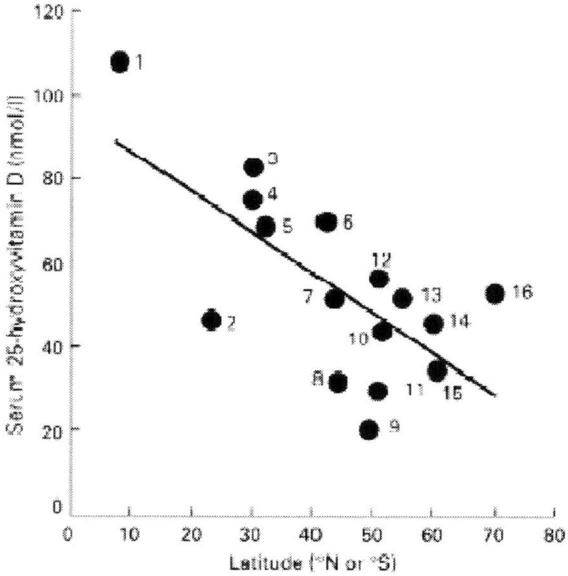

Figure 2. Mean circulating 25-hydroxyvitamin D levels in children, adolescents, and adults according to geographic latitude (r=0.68, P=0.01). (1) Children, Linhares et al. 1984; (2) male adults, Goswami et al. 2000; (3) male adolescents and adults, Looker et al. 2002; (4) female adolescents and adults, Looker et al. 2002; (5) male adults, Looker et al. 2002; (6) adolescents and adults, Tangpricha et al. 2002; (7) adults, Vieth et al. 2001; (8) children, Docio et al. 1998; (9) adolescents, Guillement et al. 2001; (10) children, Zittermann, 1987; (11) adults, Zittermann et al. 1998; (12) adults, Rucker et al. 2002; (13) children, Davies et al. 1999; (14) adults, Lamberg-Allardt et al. 2001; (15) adolescents, Lehtonen-Veromaa et al. 1999; (16) adults, Vik et al. 1980. Adopted with permission from Zittermann A," Putting cardiovascular disease and vitamin D insufficiency into perspective", British Journal of Nutrition 2005, volume 94(4), pages 483–492, Cambridge University press.

Vitamin D deficiency and cardiovascular risk. Several studies in large and heterogenic populations have demonstrated significant associations between vitamin D deficiency and cardiovascular risk factors. Study designs were both cross-sectional and prospective cohort. The association was, however, demonstrated in different cutoffs of what the authors took as being the normal range of vitamin D levels. Since some of these studies divided their population by quartiles or quintiles of vitamin D levels [4, 7] while other used a pre-specified cutoff [5, 15], the ability to define a cardiovascular protective vitamin D level to be recommended was limited. Although the definition of vitamin D deficiency varies between authors, most experts agree that >30ng/mL is optimal for adults [30, 81]. However, considering serum vitamin D levels >30ng/mL as being adequate would probably categorized the majority of individuals in the general population as being vitamin D insufficient or deficient [82]. The optimal vitamin D level for CVD health remains undetermined [83, 84], in clear contrast to the previous recommendations based on levels needed to maintain optimum bone health and prevent rickets [21]. It is therefore unknown whether these recommended values of vitamin D actually represent the levels that may be necessary to minimize the prevalence of CVD and its risk factors.

Martins et al [4] examined the association between vitamin D levels and CVD risk factors in American adults by sampling data from the Third National Health and Nutrition Examination Survey (NHANES) conducted between 1988-1994 on 7186 males and 7902 females who were ≥20 years of age. The mean vitamin D level in the overall sample was 30 ng/mL, and was lower in females, elderly persons, ethnic minorities, and participants with obesity, hypertension, and diabetes mellitus. The adjusted prevalence of hypertension, diabetes mellitus, obesity and high serum triglyceride levels was significantly higher in the first quartile of serum Vitamin D than in the fourth quartile. A follow-up report by Kim et al [3] in adults with CVD took data from fourth NHANES conducted between 2001 to 2004. Serum Vitamin D levels in that analysis, however, were divided into three categories (>30, 20-29, and <20 ng/ml), and hypovitaminosis D was defined as vitamin D <30 ng/ml. Of the 8,351 adults whose 25(OH)D was measured, the mean vitamin D level was 24.3 ng/ml, and the prevalence of hypovitaminosis D was 74%. The burden of CVD disease, i.e., prevalence of CHD, heart failure, stroke and peripheral arterial disease, increased with lower vitamin D categories. CVD was more prevalent in individuals with cardiovascular risk factors, those with CHD, and those with both CHD and heart failure after controlling for age, race, and gender when compared with persons at low risk for these factors. European populations have shown similar trends as well. Kilkkinen et al [7] showed an increased prevalence of CVD risk in the Mini-Finland Health Survey that included 6,219 males and females aged above 30 years who were free from CVD at baseline. Vitamin D levels were determined from serum collected at baseline and showed that the lowest quintile had an increased prevalence of diabetes, hypertension, inactive lifestyle, higher levels of triglycerides and lower levels of high-density lipoproteins (HDL). Steinvil et al [27] performed a cross-sectional analysis of a large ethnically diverse database derived from a Israeli health care maintenance organization. The population consisted of 34,874 individuals (76% female) aged ≥18 years, who had undergone blood tests for vitamin D levels for any reason during 2001-2008: the mean vitamin D level was 23.2 ng/ml and 22.7 ng/ml, respectively. The prevalence of vitamin D deficiency or insufficiency (vitamin D levels <30 ng/mL) for the entire study population was surprisingly high for males and females (79.2% and 77.5%, respectively), and these findings remained consistent when stratified by age. Comparing a pre-specified cut-off group of <15 ng/ml to a group with vitamin D levels >30 ng/mL, the former had higher prevalence of hypertension, diabetes mellitus, dyslipidemia, obesity and peripheral vascular disease for females and the presence of all the above except hypertension for males. Similarly, Anderson et al [85] analyzed a large electronic medical records database to determine the prevalence of vitamin D deficiency and the relation of vitamin D levels to prevalent and incident CVD risk factors. The database contained the records of 41,504 patients. The prevalence of vitamin D deficiency (<30 ng/ml) was 63.6%, with only minor differences by gender or age. Vitamin D deficiency was associated with highly significant ($p < 0.0001$) increases in the prevalence of diabetes, hypertension, hyperlipidemia, and peripheral vascular disease. Also, individuals without risk factors but with severe vitamin D deficiency had an increased likelihood of developing diabetes, hypertension, and hyperlipidemia[85]. Vitamin D deficiency has been associated with insulin resistance, type 1 and 2 diabetes mellitus, and metabolic syndrome

[86, 87]. Parker et al [18] performed a systematic review and meta-analysis to assess the risk of developing cardio-metabolic disorders by comparing groups with the highest and lowest levels of vitamin D, selecting studies on adults, and looking at the effect of vitamin D levels on outcomes relating to cardio-metabolic disorders. Included were 99,745 participants from 28 studies that met the inclusion criteria. Higher levels of vitamin D among middle-aged and elderly populations were found to be associated with a substantial decrease in CVD, type 2 diabetes and metabolic syndrome. Jorde et al [88] performed a cross-sectional study at the University of Tromso, Northern Norway, on a total of 8018 nonsmoking and 2087 smoking subjects who were included in a cross-sectional study performed in 2008. After multiple adjustments, there was a significant increase in serum total cholesterol, HDL-cholesterol (HDL-c) and low-density lipoprotein-cholesterol (LDL-c), and a significant decrease in serum LDL-C/HDL-C ratio and triglycerides across increasing serum vitamin D quartiles. Although a discussion of hypertension is beyond the scope of this chapter, it should be noted that it has also been linked to vitamin D deficiency in laboratory studies [37], geographic studies[64] as well as prospective cohort follow-up studies [15, 89].

Cardiovascular morbidity and mortality. A clear association has been reported between vitamin D deficiency and CVD morbidity and mortality. Kendrick et al [90] performed a cross-sectional analysis of data from the third NHANES (1988-1994) and examined the association between serum vitamin D levels and the prevalence of CVD, defined as a composite measure inclusive of self-reported angina, myocardial infarction or stroke, in a representative population-based sample of 16,603 males and females aged ≥18 years. After multiple adjustment for age, gender, race/ethnicity, season of measurement and traditional risk factors, participants with vitamin D deficiency (defined as <20 ng/ml) had an increased risk of prevalent CVD. Utilizing the same data from the third NHANES, Melamed et al [12] showed that the lowest quartile of vitamin D levels was independently associated with all-cause mortality, although higher (p = NS) for CVD mortality. As mentioned above, a similar CVD burden was found in the fourth NAHNES by Kim et al[3] who used a vitamin D deficiency cutoff of <30 ng/ml. Increased all-cause mortality risk in a general population was also reported by Hutchinson et al [91] in the Tromso study. Giovannucci et al [6] conducted a case-control study in 18,225 males aged 40 to 75 years who were free of diagnosed CVD and who were attending the Health Professionals Follow-up Study. During 10 years of follow-up, 454 of these men developed nonfatal myocardial infarction or fatal coronary heart disease and compared to 900 controls matched for age, date of blood collection, and smoking status. Men deficient in vitamin D (defined as <15 ng/mL) were at increased risk for myocardial infarction (RR=2.4, 95% CI, 1.53-3.84, P < 0.001 for trend) compared with those considered to be sufficient in vitamin D (>30 ng/mL). This risk remained significant even after multiple adjustment for traditional risk factors and even in men with intermediate vitamin D levels. Wang et al [5] studied 1739 Framingham Offspring Study participants who had a mean age of 59 years (55% females) without prior CVD. During a mean follow-up of 5.4 years, 120 individuals developed a first cardiovascular event. Individuals with vitamin D levels <15 ng/mL had a multivariable-adjusted hazard ratio (HR) of 1.62 for (95% CI, 1.11-2.36, p=0.01) incident cardiovascular events compared with those with vitamin D levels >15 ng/mL. This effect, however, was evident in participants with hypertension, but not in those without hypertension. Pittas et al [20] conducted a systemic review and meta-analysis in order to examine the association between vitamin D status and cardio-metabolic outcomes in generally healthy adults. Lower vitamin D levels were associated with incident CVD. Dobnig et al [52] conducted a prospective cohort study of 3,258 consecutive male and female patients scheduled for coronary angiography at a single tertiary center with the main outcome measure being all-cause and cardiovascular death stratified by vitamin D levels. During a median follow-up period of 7.7 years, 737 patients (22.6%) died, including 463 deaths from cardiovascular causes. Multivariate-adjusted HR for patients in the lower two vitamin D quartiles compared with patients in the highest vitamin D quartile were higher for all-cause mortality (HR, 2.08; 95% CI, 1.60-2.70; and HR, 1.53; 95% CI, 1.17-2.01; respectively) and for cardiovascular mortality (HR, 2.22; 95% CI, 1.57-3.13; and HR, 1.82; 95% CI, 1.29-2.58; respectively) (Figure 3).

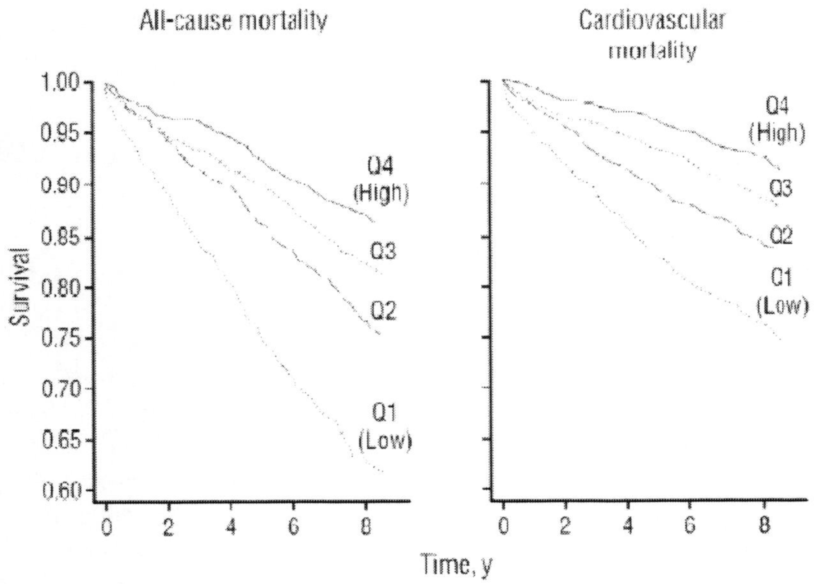

Figure 3. Kaplan-Meier plots of all-cause and cardiovascular mortality in the 25-hydroxyvitamin D quartiles (Q). Log-rank test indicated a significant difference across all 25-hydroxyvitamin D quartiles (P———————————.001). Multivariate-adjusted hazard ratios for patients in the lower two 25-hydroxyvitamin D quartiles (median, 7.6 and 13.3 ng/mL) were higher for all-cause mortality (hazard ratio, 2.08; 95% confidence interval, 1.60-2.70; and hazard ratio, 1.53; 95% confidence interval, 1.17-2.01; respectively) and for cardiovascular mortality (hazard ratio, 2.22; 95% confidence interval, 1.57-3.13; and hazard ratio, 1.82; 95% confidence interval, 1.29-2.58; respectively) compared with patients in the highest 25-hydroxyvitamin D quartile (median, 28.4 ng/mL). To convert 25-hydroxyvitamin D levels to nanomoles per liter, multiply by 2.496. Adopted with permission from Dobnig H et al, "Independent association of low serum 25-hydroxyvitamin D and 1,25-dihydroxyvitamin D levels with all-cause and cardiovascular mortality", Archives of Internal medicine 2008, volume 168(12), pages 1340-1349. Copyright© (2008) American medical Association. All rights reserved.

As mentioned earlier, Kilkkinen et al [7] conducted a prospective study based on the Mini-Finland Health Survey. After adjustment for potential confounders, the HR for total CVD death was 0.76 (95% CI, 0.60-0.95) for the highest quintile vitamin D level compared to the lowest. The association however, was evident for cerebrovascular death but not for coronary death. Pilz et al[9, 92] performed a prospective cohort study on 3,316 patients who were referred to coronary angiography between 1997 and 2000 (the Ludwigshafen Risk and Cardiovascular Health Study). During a median follow-up time of ~8 years, low levels of vitamin D were independently predictive for fatal strokes, myocardial dysfunction, deaths due to heart failure, and sudden cardiac death. Joergensen et al [93] carried out a longitudinal observational follow-up study on 289 type 2 diabetic patients who were followed for a median of 15.0 years. Their results also showed an increased risk for all-cause and cardiovascular mortality associated with severe vitamin D deficiency defined as the lower 10th percentile. This association persisted even after adjustment to multiple traditional risk factors. Refuting those findings, Jassal et al [94] conducted the only investigation on the association between vitamin D and cardiovascular mortality in a temperate climate. In their study, 1,073 Caucasian, middle-income, community-dwelling older adults living in southern California were evaluated between 1997-1999 and followed up to 10.4 (mean 6.4) years. After adjusting for age alone as well as for multiple covariates, there was no significant association between vitamin D level and cardiovascular mortality.

Vitamin D Supplementation and Cardiovascular Disease Prevention

The overwhelming evidence linking vitamin D metabolism to cardiovascular pathophysiology and demonstrating the association between its deficiency in diverse human populations, together with the increased prevalence for CVD risk factors, CVD morbidity and mortality, has propelled several randomized and controlled Vitamin D supplementation trials with the intent to prevent the often devastating outcomes of cardiovascular pathologies.

The largest trial to date was conducted by Hsia et al [19] who evaluated the risk of coronary and cerebrovascular events in the Women's Health Initiative randomized trial of calcium plus vitamin D supplementation. A total of 36,282 generally healthy postmenopausal women (50 to 79 years of age) were randomized at 40 clinical sites to calcium carbonate 500 mg with vitamin D 200 IU twice daily or to placebo. During 7 years of follow-up, calcium/vitamin D supplementation neither increased nor decreased coronary or cerebrovascular risk. Several meta-analyses were conducted on trials that examined vitamin D supplementation and its effect on all-cause and cardiovascular mortality and cardiovascular outcomes. Autier and Gandini [16] examined the risk of dying from any cause in subjects who participated in randomized trials on the impact of vitamin D supplementation. Those authors identified 18 independent randomized controlled trials that involved 57,311 participants. The summary relative risk for mortality from any cause was statistically marginal (0.93 [0.87-0.99] at 95% confidence interval), partly by decreasing CVD deaths (Figure 4).

The specific causes of prevented deaths, however, were unclear. Most trials included in that meta-analysis were conducted on frail elderly patients with a high risk for falls or fractures, and many of them had low concentrations of vitamin D and might therefore benefit from vitamin D supplementation. Pittas et al [20] examined the association between vitamin D status, including the effect of vitamin D supplementation, and cardio-metabolic outcomes in generally healthy adults. Included were 13 observational studies (14 cohorts) and 18 randomized controlled trials.

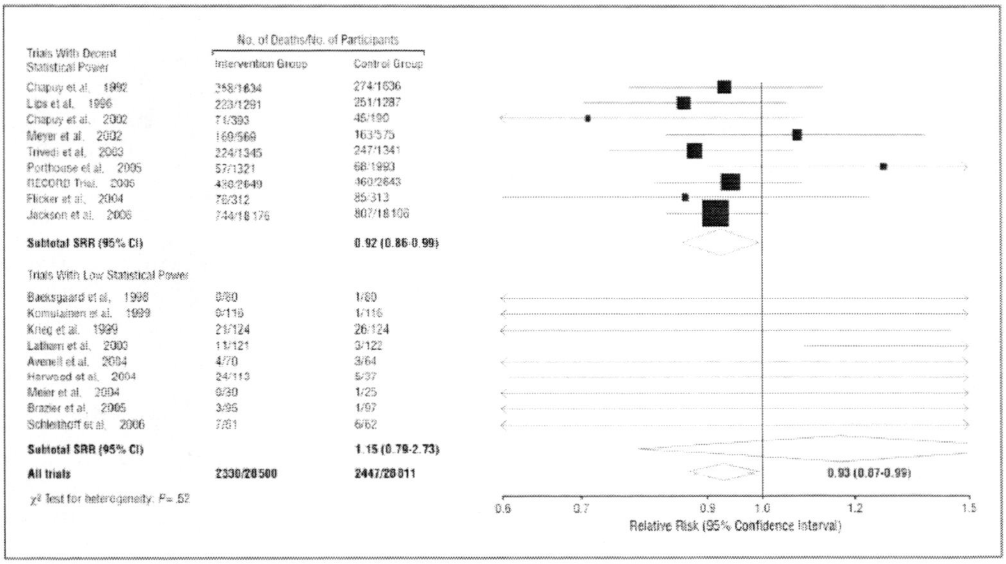

Figure 4. Meta-analysis of data on all-cause mortality in 18 randomized controlled trials with vitamin D. SRR indicates summary relative risk. Adopted with permission from Autier P. et al, "Vitamin D supplementation and total mortality: a meta-analysis of randomized controlled trials", Archives of Internal Medicine 2007, volume 67(16), pages 1730-1737. Copyright© (2007) American medical Association. All rights reserved.

Eight trials found no effect of vitamin D supplementation on glycemia or incident diabetes. In a meta-analysis of 3 cohorts studies, a lower vitamin D level was associated with incident hypertension, but supplementation did not significantly reduce systolic blood pressure or affect diastolic blood pressure in meta-analyses of 10 trials. Although the vitamin D levels were associated with incident CVD in 6 cohorts, 4 trials found no effect of supplementation on cardiovascular outcomes. Wang et al [17] performed a similar meta-analysis on 17 prospective studies and randomized trials that examined vitamin D supplementation, calcium supplementation, or both and subsequent cardiovascular events. Five prospective studies of patients receiving dialysis and 1 study involving a general population showed consistent reductions in CVD mortality among adults who received vitamin D supplements. Four prospective studies of initially healthy persons found no differences in the incidence of CVD between calcium supplement recipients and non-recipients. Results of secondary analyses in 8 randomized trials showed a slight but non-significant reduction in CVD risk.

Conclusion

The risk of cardiovascular disease, cardiovascular morbidity and cardiovascular mortality have been associated with vitamin D deficiency in numerous trials conducted on diverse populations and in geographic settings with varying amounts of solar exposure. Vitamin D has pluripotent effects on the cardiovascular system, but its cardio-protective role has yet to be defined. Vitamin D deficiency might reflect a lack of sun exposure, therefore raising the possibility that it could be a biomarker of an essentially indoor lifestyle rather than the cause of increased CVD risk [1]. Despite the promise for disease prevention suggested by many published studies, the evidence for widespread use of high-dose vitamin D supplementation for the prevention of CVD events in the general population remains inconclusive [22].

Conducting large randomized trials of high-dose vitamin D supplementation in general population settings is warranted. There is a need for a better definition of the optimal dose, the real benefits, and the potentially harmful effects of vitamin D supplementation, as well as for the possible harm of lower ranges of vitamin D levels on human health.

References

[1] Lee JH, O'Keefe JH, Bell D, Hensrud DD and Holick MF. Vitamin D deficiency an important, common, and easily treatable cardiovascular risk factor? *Journal of the American College of Cardiology* 2008;52:1949-56.

[2] Wallis DE, Penckofer S and Sizemore GW. The "sunshine deficit" and cardiovascular disease. *Circulation* 2008;118:1476-85.

[3] Kim DH, Sabour S, Sagar UN, Adams S and Whellan DJ. Prevalence of hypovitaminosis D in cardiovascular diseases (from the National Health and Nutrition Examination Survey 2001 to 2004). *The American journal of cardiology* 2008;102:1540-4.

[4] Martins D, Wolf M, Pan D, Zadshir A, Tareen N, Thadhani R *et al.* Prevalence of cardiovascular risk factors and the serum levels of 25-hydroxyvitamin D in the United States: data from the Third National Health and Nutrition Examination Survey. *Archives of internal medicine* 2007;167:1159-65.

[5] Wang TJ, Pencina MJ, Booth SL, Jacques PF, Ingelsson E, Lanier K *et al.* Vitamin D deficiency and risk of cardiovascular disease. *Circulation* 2008;117:50.11-3

[6] Giovannucci E, Liu Y, Hollis BW and Rimm EB. 25-hydroxyvitamin D and risk of myocardial infarction in men: a prospective study. *Archives of internal medicine* 2008;168:1174-80.

[7] Kilkkinen A, Knekt P, Aro A, Rissanen H, Marniemi J, Heliovaara M *et al.* Vitamin D Status and the Risk of Cardiovascular Disease Death. *American journal of epidemiology* 2009.

[8] Scragg R, Jackson R, Holdaway IM, Lim T and Beaglehole R. Myocardial infarction is inversely associated with plasma 25-hydroxyvitamin D3 levels: a community-based study. *International journal of epidemiology* 1990;19:559-63.

[9] Pilz S, Dobnig H, Fischer JE, Wellnitz B, Seelhorst U, Boehm BO *et al.* Low vitamin d levels predict stroke in patients referred to coronary angiography. *Stroke; a journal of cerebral circulation* 2008;39:2611-3.

[10] Poole KE, Loveridge N, Barker PJ, Halsall DJ, Rose C, Reeve J *et al.* Reduced vitamin D in acute stroke. *Stroke; a journal of cerebral circulation* 2006;37:243-5.

[11] Zittermann A, Schleithoff SS, Tenderich G, Berthold HK, Korfer R and Stehle P. Low vitamin D status: a contributing factor in the pathogenesis of congestive heart failure? *Journal of the American College of Cardiology* 2003;41:105-12.

[12] Melamed ML, Muntner P, Michos ED, Uribarri J, Weber C, Sharma J *et al* .Serum 25-hydroxyvitamin D levels and the prevalence of peripheral arterial disease: results from

NHANES 2001 to 2004. *Arteriosclerosis, thrombosis, and vascular biology* 2008;28:1179-85.

[13] Gaddipati VC, Kuriacose R, Copeland R, Bailey BA and Peiris AN. Vitamin D deficiency: an increasing concern in peripheral arterial disease. *J. Am. Med. Dir. Assoc.* 2010;11:308-11.

[14] Scragg R, Sowers M and Bell C. Serum 25-hydroxyvitamin D, diabetes, and ethnicity in the Third National Health and Nutrition Examination Survey *.Diabetes care* 2004;27:2813-8.

[15] Forman JP, Giovannucci E, Holmes MD, Bischoff-Ferrari HA, Tworoger SS, Willett WC *et al.* Plasma 25-hydroxyvitamin D levels and risk of incident hypertension. *Hypertension* 2007;49:1063-9.

[16] Autier P and Gandini S. Vitamin D supplementation and total mortality: a meta-analysis of randomized controlled trials. *Archives of internal medicine* 2007;167:1730-7.

[17] Wang L, Manson JE, Song Y and Sesso HD. Systematic review: vitamin d and calcium supplementation in prevention of cardiovascular events. *Annals of internal medicine* 2010;152:315-23.

[18] Parker J, Hashmi O, Dutton D, Mavrodaris A, Stranges S, Kandala NB *et al.* Levels of vitamin D and cardiometabolic disorders: systematic review and meta-analysis. *Maturitas* 2010;65:225-36.

[19] Hsia J, Heiss G, Ren H, Allison M, Dolan NC, Greenland P *et al.* Calcium/vitamin D supplementation and cardiovascular events. *Circulation* 2007;115:846-54.

[20] Pittas AG, Chung M, Trikalinos T, Mitri J, Brendel M, Patel K *et al.* Systematic review: Vitamin D and cardiometabolic outcomes. *Annals of internal medicine* 2010;152:307-14.

[21] Rao D, Villanueva A and Mathews M. Histologic evolution of vitamin depletion in patients with intestinal malabsorption or dietary deficiency. In: Frame B, Potts JT, eds. Clinical Disorders of Bone and Mineral Metabolism. Amsterdam, the Netherlands:Excerpta Medica; 1983:321-330.

[22] Guallar E, Miller ER, 3rd, Ordovas JM and Stranges S. Vitamin D supplementation in the age of lost innocence. *Annals of internal medicine* 2010; 19-52:327.

[23] O'Connell TD, Berry JE, Jarvis AK, Somerman MJ and Simpson RU. 1,25-Dihydroxyvitamin D3 regulation of cardiac myocyte proliferation and hypertrophy. *Am. J. Physiol.* 1997;272:H1751-8.

[24] Forman JP, Williams JS and Fisher ND. Plasma 25-hydroxyvitamin D and regulation of the renin-angiotensin system in humans. *Hypertension* 2010;55:1283-8.

[25] Canning MO GK, de Wit H, Ruwhof C, Drexhage HA. 1-alpha,25-Dihydroxyvitamin D3 (1,25(OH)(2)D(3)) hampers the maturation of fully active immature dendritic cells from monocytes. *Eur. J. Endocrinol.* 2001;145:351–7.

[26] Wang TJ, Zhang F, Richards JB, Kestenbaum B, van Meurs JB, Berry D *et al.* Common genetic determinants of vitamin D insufficiency: a genome-wide association study. *Lancet* 2010;376:180-8.

[27] Steinvil A ,Leshem-Rubinow E, Berliner S, Justo D, Finn T, Ish-Shalom M *et al.* Vitamin D deficiency prevalence and cardiovascular risk in Israel. *European journal of clinical investigation* 2010.

[28] Simpson RU and Weishaar RE. Involvement of 1,25-dihydroxyvitamin D3 in regulating myocardial calcium metabolism: physiological and pathological actions. *Cell Calcium* 1988;9:285-92.

[29] Walters MR. Newly identified actions of the vitamin D endocrine system. *Endocr. Rev.* 1992;13:719-64.

[30] Holick MF. Vitamin D deficiency. *The New England journal of medicine* 2007;357:266-81.

[31] Nagpal S, Na S and Rathnachalam R. Noncalcemic actions of vitamin D receptor ligands. *Endocr. Rev.* 2005;26:662-87.

[32] Holick MF, Garabedian M. Vitamin D: photobiology, metabolism, mechanism of action, and clinical applications. In: Favus MJ, ed. Primer on the metabolic bone diseases and disorders of mineral metabolism. 6th ed. Washington, DC: American Society for Bone and Mineral research, 2006:129-37.

[33] Bachschmid MM and van der Loo B. A new "sunshine" in the vasculature? *Circulation* 2005;111:1571-3.

[34] Weishaar RE and Simpson RU. Involvement of vitamin D3 with cardiovascular function. II. Direct and indirect effects. *Am. J. Physiol.* 1987;253:E675-83.

[35] O'Connell TD, Giacherio DA, Jarvis AK and Simpson RU .Inhibition of cardiac myocyte maturation by 1,25-dihydroxyvitamin D3. *Endocrinology* 1995;136:482-8.

[36] Chen S, Glenn DJ, Ni W, Grigsby CL, Olsen K, Nishimoto M *et al.* Expression of the Vitamin D Receptor Is Increased in the Hypertrophic Heart. *Hypertension* 2008;52:1106-12.

[37] Xiang W, Kong J, Chen S, Cao LP, Qiao G, Zheng W *et al.* Cardiac hypertrophy in vitamin D receptor knockout mice: role of the systemic and cardiac renin-angiotensin systems. *Am. J. Physiol. Endocrinol. Metab.* 2005;288:E125-32.

[38] Somjen D ,Weisman Y, Kohen F, Gayer B, Limor R, Sharon O *et al.* 25-hydroxyvitamin D3-1alpha-hydroxylase is expressed in human vascular smooth muscle cells and is upregulated by parathyroid hormone and estrogenic compounds. *Circulation* 2005;111:1666-71.

[39] Merke J ,Hofmann W, Goldschmidt D and Ritz E. Demonstration of 1,25(OH)2 vitamin D3 receptors and actions in vascular smooth muscle cells in vitro. *Calcif Tissue Int.* 1987;41:112-4.

[40] Merke J, Milde P, Lewicka S, Hugel U, Klaus G, Mangelsdorf DJ *et al.* Identification and regulation of 1,25-dihydroxyvitamin D3 receptor activity and biosynthesis of 1,25-dihydroxyvitamin D3. Studies in cultured bovine aortic endothelial cells and human dermal capillaries. *J. Clin. Invest.* 1989;83:1903-15.

[41] Davies MR HK. Pathophysiological mechanisms of vascular calcification in end-stage renal disease.. *Kidney int.* 2001;60:472-9.

[42] Watson KE, Abrolat ML, Malone LL, Hoeg JM, Doherty T, Detrano R *et al.* Active serum vitamin D levels are inversely correlated with coronary calcification. *Circulation* 1997;96:1755-60.

[43] London GM, Guerin AP, Verbeke FH, Pannier B, Boutouyrie P, Marchais SJ *et al.* Mineral metabolism and arterial functions in end-stage renal disease: potential role of 25-hydroxyvitamin D deficiency. *J. Am. Soc. Nephrol.* 2007.20-18:613;

[44] Matias PJ, Ferreira C, Jorge C, Borges M, Aires I, Amaral T *et al.* 25-Hydroxyvitamin D3, arterial calcifications and cardiovascular risk markers in haemodialysis patients. *Nephrol. Dial Transplant* 2009;24:611-8.

[45] Dong Y, Stallmann-Jorgensen IS, Pollock NK, Harris RA, Keeton D, Huang Y *et al.* A 16-week randomized clinical trial of 2000 international units daily vitamin D3 supplementation in black youth: 25-hydroxyvitamin D, adiposity, and arterial stiffness. *The Journal of clinical endocrinology and metabolism* 2010;95:4584-91.

[46] Garcia-Canton C, Bosch E, Ramirez A, Gonzalez Y, Auyanet I, Guerra R *et al.* Vascular calcification and 25-hydroxyvitamin D levels in non-dialysis patients with chronic kidney disease stages 4 and 5. *Nephrol. Dial Transplant* 2010.

[47] Zittermann A, Schleithoff SS and Koerfer R. Putting cardiovascular disease and vitamin D insufficiency into perspective. *Br. J. Nutr.* 2005;94:483-92.

[48] Chen S, Nakamura K and Gardner DG. 1,25-dihydroxyvitamin D inhibits human ANP gene promoter activity. *Regul. Pept.* 2005;128:197-202.

[49] Wu J, Garami M, Cao L, Li Q and Gardner DG. 1,25(OH)2D3 suppresses expression and secretion of atrial natriuretic peptide from cardiac myocytes. *Am. J. Physiol.* 1995;268:E1108-13.

[50] Yee YK, Chintalacharuvu SR, Lu J and Nagpal S. Vitamin D receptor modulators for inflammation and cancer. *Mini. Rev. Med. Chem.* 2005;5:761-78.

[51] Suzuki Y, Ichiyama T, Ohsaki A, Hasegawa S, Shiraishi M and Furukawa S. Anti-inflammatory effect of 1alpha,25-dihydroxyvitamin D(3) in human coronary arterial endothelial cells: Implication for the treatment of Kawasaki disease. *J. Steroid Biochem. Mol. Biol.* 2009;113:134-8.

[52] Dobnig H, Pilz S, Scharnagl H, Renner W, Seelhorst U, Wellnitz B *et al.* Independent association of low serum 25-hydroxyvitamin d and 1,25-dihydroxyvitamin d levels with all-cause and cardiovascular mortality. *Archives of internal medicine* 2008;168:1340-9.

[53] Equils O, Naiki Y, Shapiro AM, Michelsen K, Lu D, Adams J *et al.* 1,25-Dihydroxyvitamin D inhibits lipopolysaccharide-induced immune activation in human endothelial cells. *Clin. Exp. Immunol.* 2006;143:58-64.

[54] Martinesi M, Bruni S, Stio M and Treves C. 1,25-Dihydroxyvitamin D3 inhibits tumor necrosis factor-alpha-induced adhesion molecule expression in endothelial cells. *Cell Biol. Int.* 2006;30:365-75.

[55] Muller K HP, Diamant M, Rieneck K, Kharazmi A, Bendtzen K. 1,25-Dihydroxyvitamin D3 inhibits cytokine production by human blood monocytes at the post-transcriptional level. *Cytokine* 1992;4:506-12.

[56] Inoue M, Wakasugi M, Wakao R, Gan N, Tawata M, Nishii Y *et al.* A synthetic analogue of vitamin D3, 22-oxa-1,25-dihydroxy-vitamin D3, stimulates the production of prostacyclin by vascular tissues. *Life Sciences* 1992;51:1105-12.

[57] Wakasugi M, Noguchi T, Inoue M, Kazama Y, Tawata M, Kanemaru Y *et al.* Vitamin D3 stimulates the production of prostacyclin by vascular smooth muscle cells. *Prostaglandins* 1991;42:127-36.

[58] Schluter KD and Piper HM. Cardiovascular actions of parathyroid hormone and parathyroid hormone-related peptide. *Cardiovasc Res.* 1998;37:34-41.

[59] Saleh FN, Schirmer H, Sundsfjord J and Jorde R. Parathyroid hormone and left ventricular hypertrophy. *Eur. Heart J.* 2003;24:2054-60.

[60] Hagstrom E, Hellman P, Larsson TE, Ingelsson E, Berglund L, Sundstrom J *et al.* Plasma parathyroid hormone and the risk of cardiovascular mortality in the community. *Circulation* 2009;119:2765-71.

[61] Hagstrom E, Ingelsson E, Sundstrom J, Hellman P, Larsson TE, Berglund L *et al.* Plasma parathyroid hormone and risk of congestive heart failure in the community. *Eur. J. Heart Fail* 2010;12:1186-92.

[62] Pilz S, Tomaschitz A, Drechsler C, Ritz E, Boehm BO, Grammer TB *et al.* Parathyroid hormone level is associated with mortality and cardiovascular events in patients undergoing coronary angiography. *Eur. Heart J.* 2010;31:1591-8.

[63] Cawthon PM, Parimi N, Barrett-Connor E, Laughlin GA, Ensrud KE, Hoffman AR *et al.* Serum 25-hydroxyvitamin D, parathyroid hormone, and mortality in older men. *The Journal of clinical endocrinology and metabolism* 2010;95:4625-34.

[64] Rostand SG. Ultraviolet light may contribute to geographic and racial blood pressure differences. *Hypertension* 1997;30:150-6.

[65] Fleck A. Latitude and ischaemic heart disease. *Lancet* 1989;1:613.

[66] Rich DQ, Gaziano JM and Kurth T. Geographic patterns in overall and specific cardiovascular disease incidence in apparently healthy men in the United States. *Stroke; a journal of cerebral circulation* 2007;38:2221-7.

[67] Holick M. Vitamin D: the underappreciated D-lightful hormone that is important for skeletal and cellular health. *Curr Opin Endocrinol Diabetes* 2002;9:87-98.

[68] Rigel DS, Rigel EG and Rigel AC. Effects of altitude and latitude on ambient UVB radiation. *J. Am. Acad Dermatol.* 1999;40:114-6.

[69] Mortimer EA, Jr., Monson RR and MacMahon B. Reduction in mortality from coronary heart disease in men residing at high altitude. *The New England journal of medicine* 1977;296:581-5.

[70] Gordan R and Danner R. Coronary heart disease at high altitudes. *The New England journal of medicine* 1977;297:60-2.

[71] Scragg R .Seasonality of cardiovascular disease mortality and the possible protective effect of ultra-violet radiation. *International journal of epidemiology* 1981;10:337-41.

[72] Douglas AS, Dunnigan MG, Allan TM and Rawles JM. Seasonal variation in coronary heart disease in Scotland. *J. Epidemiol. Community Health* 1995;49:575-82.

[73] Grimes DS, Hindle E and Dyer T. Respiratory infection and coronary heart disease: progression of a paradigm. *QJM* 2000;93:375-83.

[74] Spielberg C, Falkenhahn D, Willich SN, Wegscheider K and Voller H. Circadian, day-of-week, and seasonal variability in myocardial infarction: comparison between working and retired patients. *American heart journal* 1996;132:579-85.

[75] Enquselassie F, Dobson AJ, Alexander HM and Steele PL. Seasons, temperature and coronary disease. *International journal of epidemiology* 1993;22:632-6.

[76] Douglas AS, Russell D and Allan TM. Seasonal, regional and secular variations of cardiovascular and cerebrovascular mortality in New Zealand. *Aust. N. Z. J. Med.* 1990;20:669-76.

[77] Kloner RA, Poole WK and Perritt RL. When throughout the year is coronary death most likely to occur? A 12-year population-based analysis of more than 220 000 cases. *Circulation* 1999;100:1630-4.

[78] Madjid M, Naghavi M, Litovsky S and Casscells SW. Influenza and cardiovascular disease: a new opportunity for prevention and the need for further studies. *Circulation* 2003;108:2730-6.
[79] Marsden PA. Inflammation and coagulation in the cardiovascular system: the contribution of influenza. *Circ. Res.* 2006;99:1152-3.
[80] Steinvil A, Berliner S, Bromberg M, Cohen M, Shalev V, Shapira I *et al.* Micro-inflammatory changes in asymptomatic healthy adults during bouts of respiratory tract infections in the community: potential triggers for atherothrombotic events. *Atherosclerosis* 2009;206:270-5.
[81] Bischoff-Ferrari HA, Giovannucci E, Willett WC, Dietrich T and Dawson-Hughes B. Estimation of optimal serum concentrations of 25-hydroxyvitamin D for multiple health outcomes. *The American journal of clinical nutrition* 2006;84:18-28.
[82] Thomas MK, Lloyd-Jones DM, Thadhani RI, Shaw AC, Deraska DJ, Kitch BT *et al.* Hypovitaminosis D in medical inpatients. *The New England journal of medicine* 1998;338:777-83.
[83] Dawson-Hughes B, Heaney RP, Holick MF, Lips P, Meunier PJ and Vieth R. Estimates of optimal vitamin D status. *Osteoporos Int* 2005;16:713-6.
[84] Vieth R. What is the optimal vitamin D status for health? *Progress in biophysics and molecular biology* 2006;92:26-32.
[85] Anderson JL, May HT, Horne BD, Bair TL, Hall NL, Carlquist JF *et al* .Relation of vitamin D deficiency to cardiovascular risk factors, disease status, and incident events in a general healthcare population. *The American journal of cardiology* 2010;106:963-8.
[86] Hypponen E, Laara E, Reunanen A, Jarvelin MR and Virtanen SM .Intake of vitamin D and risk of type 1 diabetes: a birth-cohort study. *Lancet* 2001;358:1500-3.
[87] Pittas AG, Lau J, Hu FB and Dawson-Hughes B. The role of vitamin D and calcium in type 2 diabetes. A systematic review and meta-analysis. *The Journal of clinical endocrinology and metabolism* 2007;92:2017-29.
[88] Jorde R, Figenschau Y, Hutchinson M, Emaus N and Grimnes G. High serum 25-hydroxyvitamin D concentrations are associated with a favorable serum lipid profile. *Eur J Clin Nutr* 2010;64:1457-64.
[89] Jorde R, Figenschau Y, Emaus N, Hutchinson M and Grimnes G. Serum 25-hydroxyvitamin D levels are strongly related to systolic blood pressure but do not predict future hypertension. *Hypertension* 2010;55:792-8.
[90] Kendrick J, Targher G, Smits G and Chonchol M. 25-Hydroxyvitamin D deficiency is independently associated with cardiovascular disease in the Third National Health and Nutrition Examination Survey. *Atherosclerosis* 2009;205:255-60.
[91] Hutchinson MS, Grimnes G, Joakimsen RM, Figenschau Y and Jorde R. Low serum 25-hydroxyvitamin D levels are associated with increased all-cause mortality risk in a general population: the Tromso study. *Eur. J. Endocrinol.* 2010;162:935-42.
[92] Pilz S, Marz W, Wellnitz B, Seelhorst U, Fahrleitner-Pammer A, Dimai HP *et al.* Association of vitamin D deficiency with heart failure and sudden cardiac death in a large cross-sectional study of patients referred for coronary angiography. *The Journal of clinical endocrinology and metabolism* 2008;93:3927-35.
[93] Joergensen C, Gall MA, Schmedes A, Tarnow L, Parving HH and Rossing P. Vitamin D levels and mortality in type 2 diabetes. *Diabetes care* 2010;33:2238-43.

[94] Jassal SK, Chonchol M, von Muhlen D, Smits G and Barrett-Connor E. Vitamin d, parathyroid hormone, and cardiovascular mortality in older adults: the rancho bernardo study. *Am. J. Med.* 2010;123:1114-20.

In: Vitamin D Deficiency
Editors: V. Lerner and C. Miodownik

ISBN: 978-1-61470-964-0

Chapter V

Role of Hypovitaminosis D in Osteoporotic Hip Fracture

Marta Larrosa**, Enrique Casado and Ivonne Vázquez
Hospital of Sabadell. Corporació Sanitària i Universitària Parc Taulí (UAB).
Sabadell (Barcelona), Spain

Abstract

Hip fracture (HF) is the osteoporotic fracture with higher socioeconomic costs and higher morbidity and mortality. HF mainly affects elderly women, and its incidence increases exponentially with age. Although HF is usually considered as a homogeneous condition, there are two main types of HF according to the involved anatomic site: fractures of the femoral neck (intracapsular fractures) and fractures of the intertrochanteric region (extracapsular fractures). Patients with intertrochanteric fractures tend to be older, thinner, have lower bone mineral density (BMD) and suffer more previous osteoporotic fractures than patients with intracapsular fractures. Hypovitaminosis D is highly prevalent among patients with HF, being serum 25(OH)D levels low and similar between patients with cervical and intertrochanteric HF. The overall prevalence of secondary hyperparathyroidism due to hypovitaminosis D in patients with HF is about 35-50%, and it is a strong independent predictor of poor outcome. Patients with extracapsular fractures have a significantly higher prevalence of secondary hyperparathyroidism and show significantly higher levels of serum PTH. Serum 25(OH)D levels are associated with the risk of HF. Several factors are associated with hypovitaminosis D development, such as advancing age, lack of physical activity, co-morbidities and frailty, low sun exposition, undernutrition or low functional status.

There is a clear seasonal incidence of HF, with the highest incidence observed in winter and the lowest in summer, when patients have higher 25(OH)D3 levels and lower PTH levels. Some authors have found an inverse correlation between the monthly number of fractures and 25(OH)D3 serum levels, and a direct correlation between

* Corresponding author: Marta Larrosa Padro, MD, PhD. Chief of Rheumatology Service, Hospital of Sabadell, Rheumatology Department, Corporació Sanitària i Universitària Parc Taulí (UAB), Parc Tauli s/n, 08208 Sabadell (Barcelona), Spain. Phone: +34937231010;Fax +34937160646 E-mail: mlarrosa@tauli.cat.

25(OH)D3 serum levels and the average solar radiation during the 2nd and 3rd previous month.

Vitamin D deficiency has been shown to be associated with some degree of myopathy and falls, and with HF severity, so the more severe HF, such as displaced femoral neck fractures and unstable intertrochanteric fractures are more frequent among patients with low vitamin D levels. Although a daily vitamin D oral supplementation with cholecalciferol seems to reduce the risk of hip and any non-vertebral fractures, there is an insufficient prescription of calcium and vitamin D supplements in these patients. Probably, vitamin D supplementation strategies using an easy posology with a wider interval of administration (weekly or monthly) could be more appropriate to optimize the individual adherence of these patients.

Keywords: Hip fracture; Vitamin D; 25(OH)D; Risk factors

Abbreviations

HF	Hip fracture
OP	Osteoporosis
BMD	Bone Mineral Density
BMI	Body Mass index
CI	Confidence interval
RR	Relative risk
OR	Odds ratio

Introduction

Hip fracture (HF) is the most serious of all osteoporotic fractures. Among osteoporotic fractures HF is the one associated with the most important morbidity and mortality [1-5] and higher socioeconomic costs [6], representing a major health problem in developed countries. Mortality is about 30% in the first year after the fracture, and life expectancy is reduced about 9 years. One-third of previously independent patients become totally dependent and half partly dependent [1].

HF mainly affects elderly women and is the most frequent fracture after the age of 75. Its incidence increases exponentially with age so that by the ninth decade of life, it is estimated that 1 in 3 women and 1 in 6 men will suffer a HF [7]. Population aging has led to an increase in the crude incidence of HF over the second half of the 20th century [8, 9], and with life expectancy rising worldwide, the incidence of HF in elderly individuals is estimated to rise from 1.66 million in 1990 to 6.26 million in 2050 [10].

The epidemiology of HF has been widely analyzed in numerous countries and notable differences in incidence rates have been found among different continents, different countries and even among different regions of the same country. Rates are highest in countries of Northern Europe and in United States, intermediate in Asian populations, and lowest in Latin America and African countries [11]. Among different ethnic populations, the highest fracture rates are seen in Caucasians and the lowest in black patients, both native African and Afro-

Americans. There is also a north-south gradient, particularly in Europe, where more hip fractures occur in north Europe compared to the south [9, 11, 12]. The reasons for these geographic and ethnic variations are not well understood, although genetic and environmental factors could play a role. In fact, environmental factors such as type of diet and vitamin D status are recognised as important factors in the pathogenesis of these fractures.

The presentation of HF seems to have gradually evolved in recent decades. It has been observed an increase in the age of patients, so that the average age in the current series is over 80 years while in the series published in the 80's the average age was around 79 years [13, 14] and in the 40's around 67 years [15].

Even though crude incidence of HF in the elderly is increasing because of population aging, age-adjusted incidence rates have stabilized in some countries. In this sense epidemiological studies in the United States and some European countries show a stabilization and even a slight decrease in the incidence of age-adjusted HF in recent last years [9, 16-18]. This fact may be attributable to a better health status among elderly people, and the success of osteoporosis prevention and treatment programs.

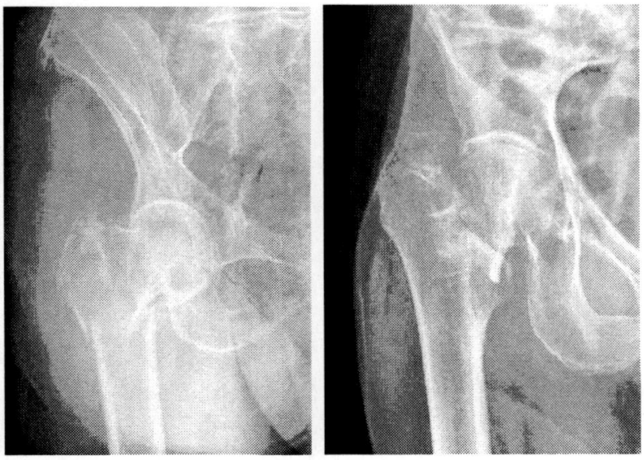

Figure 1. A. Subtrochanteric fracture. B. Basicervical fracture.

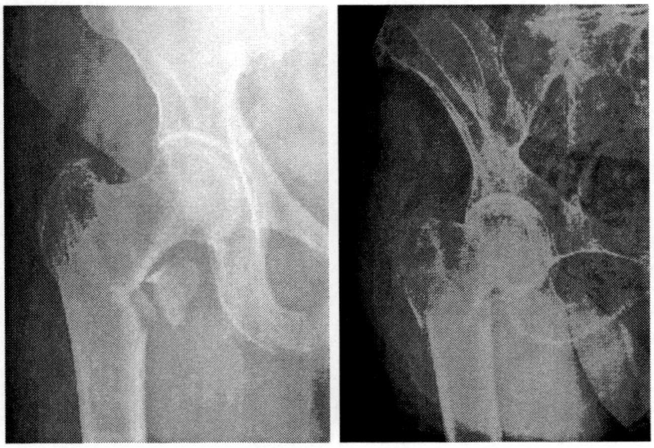

Figure 2. A. Interthrochanteric fracture. B. Subtrochanteric fracture.

Although HF is usually considered in most studies as a homogeneous condition, there are two main types of hip fracture according to the involved anatomic site: fractures of the femoral neck (intracapsular fractures) and fractures of the intertrochanteric region (extracapsular fractures), that can have different characteristics and different outcomes. The intracapsular fractures include subcapital, and basicervical varieties (figure 1); and extracapsular fractures include intertrochanteric and subtrochanteric fractures (figure 2). Subcapital and intertrochanteric fractures account for more than 90% of HF.

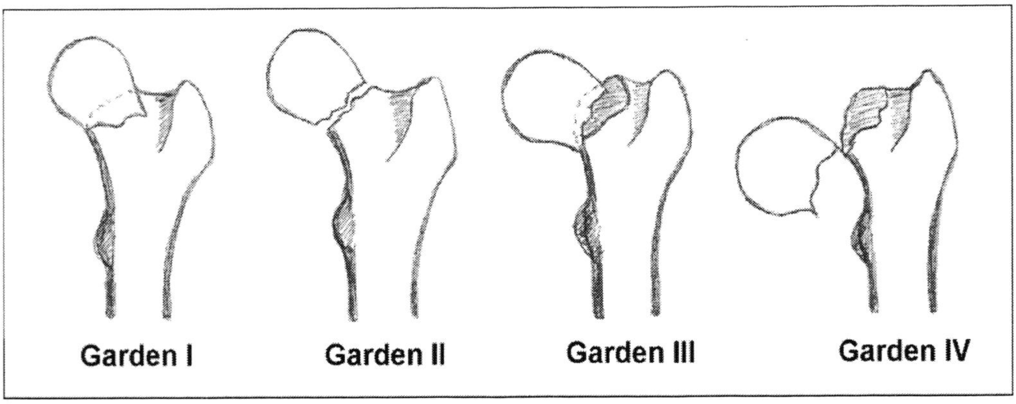

Figure 3. Femoral neck fractures according to Garden classification. Garden I: Incomplete or impacted fracture, in which bone structure is preserved at the bottom of the femoral neck. Garden II: Complete fracture without displacement of fragments. Garden III: Complete fracture with partial displacement of the bone fragments. Garden IV: Complete fracture with total displacement of the bone fragments.

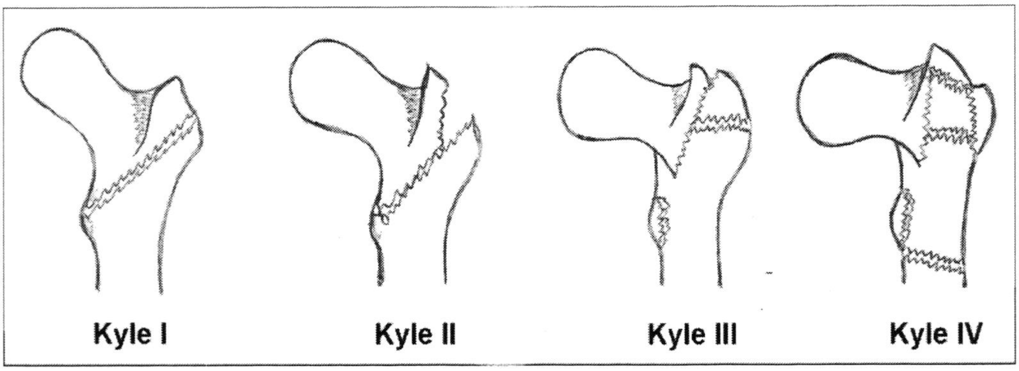

Figure 4. Intertrochanteric fractures according to Kyle classification: Kyle I. A single fracture line without displacement of the two fragments. Kyle II: Stable fracture with displaced varus proximal fragment and minimal comminution. Kyle III: Unstable fracture with displaced varus proximal fragment. Kyle IV: Similar to Kyle III but with extension of the fracture at the subtrochanteric region.

The Garden staging system [19] is used to classify femoral neck fractures (figure 3), while Kyle classification can be used to classify intertrochanteric fractures according to fragmentation and displacement (figure 4) [20].

More severe HF such as displaced femoral neck fractures (Garden III and IV) and unstable intertrochanteric fractures (Kyle III and IV) lead to poor outcomes.

Differences between Neck and Trochanteric HF

The trochanteric region has a 50% proportion of trabecular bone compared with the 25% of the femoral neck [21]. An age-related deterioration in the microarquitecture of the femoral subregions (medial neck, lateral neck, and intertrochanteric region) has been described for both genders. However trabecular deterioration is most significant in the intertrochanteric region in women, while the lateral neck is the most affected in men [22]. Given these differences in bone composition between both regions, it is possible to hypothesize a different aetiology, different risk factors and different pathogenic mechanisms of the fracture.

The characteristics of patients may also differ between femoral neck and intertrochanteric fractures. Some studies suggest that patients with fracture of the trochanteric region are older [23, 24], with a female:male ratio similar in both groups (3:1), and without differences in socio-demographic, number of comorbidities, life-style habits and functional status [23, 24]. Regarding haematological or biochemical variables, only haemoglobin and albumin levels [24] or total lymphocyte count [23] were slightly lower in patients with intertrochanteric fractures. Although the length of hospital stay and functional outcome are similar between patients with cervical or trochanteric HF [24, 25], the in-hospital mortality rate has been described as being higher among patients with trochanteric fractures [25-28], albeit not confirmed by Fisher et al [24].

Some authors have shown that women with intertrochanteric fractures are thinner [29] and often had suffered previous osteoporotic fractures compared with patients with intracapsular fractures [23].

Bone mineral density (BMD) seems to be significantly lower in women with intertrochanteric fractures compared with those with femoral neck fractures [30, 31]. Regarding geometrical, structural, and mechanical characteristics of the proximal femur some significant differences have also been found between patients with cervical and intertrochanteric HF [32-36].

Prevalence of Hypovitaminosis D in HF

Hypovitaminosis D is common among older adults especially during winter, in medical inpatients [37], and especially highly prevalent in nursing home residents [38, 39] and patients with HF.

A high prevalence of low serum 25(OH)D among HF patients and the importance of vitamin D insufficiency in the pathogenesis of the fracture was first described 30 years ago [40, 41]. The prevalence of hypovitaminosis D among patients with HF has been studied in different countries, mainly in Europe and in the United States, showing some differences: 36%-53% in Finland [42-44], 50% in USA [45], 40%-81% in United Kingdom [41, 46, 47], 80% in Switzerland [48], 67%-91% in Spain [38, 49], 65% in Russia, [50]. This prevalence may be variable depending on whether the population is analyzed throughout the year or only during a certain season, if the population analyzed is from the same or different latitude, and of course depending on the 25(OH)D levels used to define vitamin D deficiency. Time of blood extraction is also very important, since just 24 hours after a fracture or after a significant surgical procedure some plasma components, like albumin decrease [51].

Subsequently vitamin D metabolites (Vitamin D-binding Protein, 25(OH)D and 24,25$(OH)_2$D) [52] also decrease and could alter the real prevalence of hypovitaminosis D and could make difficult to compare different series. Serum 25(OH)D levels are low and similar between patients with cervical and intertrochanteric HF [23, 24] and the prevalence of hypovitaminosis D (25(OH)D <20 ng /ml), and vitamin D deficiency (25(OH)D <10 ng /ml) did not differ significantly between both groups [24].

Hipovitaminosis D and Secondary Hyperparathyroidism

The parathyroid hormone-vitamin D system is a major regulator of bone metabolism and mineral homeostasis, and controls the concentration of serum calcium through its effects on gut, kidney and bone. In hypovitaminosis D there is a decrease in the intestinal absorption of calcium and a subsequent decrease in serum calcium levels. This relative hypocalcemia stimulates parathyroid hormone (PTH) secretion (secondary hyperparathyroidism), which enhances the levels of renal 1-α-hydroxylase and 1,25$(OH)_2$D, leading to an increase of calcium absorption and the maintenance of the calcium homeostasis. However, this secondary hyperparathyroidism leads to a high bone turn-over, with an excess of bone resorption over formation, resulting in a progressive bone loss [46, 53].

The overall prevalence of secondary hyperparathyroidism due to hypovitaminosis D in patients with HF is about 35-50% [23, 27, 46, 54], similar to that observed in a matched population of hospitalized older patients with hypovitaminosis D, but without HF [54]. In fact, the presence of secondary hyperparathyroidism among patients with HF does not imply to have different demographic characteristics or different functional capacity previous to the fracture [23, 46]. Patients with hypovitaminosis D and with normal PTH levels may have some degree of "functional hypoparathyroidism", that could explain this inappropriate low level of parathyroid hormone [46]. Patients with hypovitaminosis D usually show levels of calcium and 1,25$(OH)_2$D within the normal range but significantly lower than vitamin D-replete patients. These levels of 1,25-$(OH)_2$D are significantly lower in patients with hypovitaminosis D without hyperparathyroidism, compared with subjects with hypovitaminosis D and secondary hyperparathyroidism, suggesting a failure of the parathyroid gland to mount and adequate parathyroid hormone response. However, the low 1,25-$(OH)_2$D levels observed in patients with hypovitaminosis D, with or without secondary hyperparathyroidism, could be also explained by other factors, as an impaired 1-α-hydroxylation of an ageing kidney, even though a normal function [55]. PTH levels sufficient to produce bone mineral abnormalities remains to be defined as well as the arbitrary definition of secondary hyperparathyroidism (serum PTH level above the standard laboratory reference range), that may vary between different laboratories. Despite the fact that low 25(OH)D levels are similar among patients with cervical and intertrochanteric HF [23, 24], the presence and severity of secondary hyperparathyroidism is different between them. Patients with extracapsular fracture have a significantly higher prevalence of secondary hyperparathyroidism (41-60% vs 30-47%) and show significantly higher levels of serum PTH [23, 24, 27]. Also phosphate levels are higher among patients with HF compared with controls [56], although only in patients with extracapsular fracture these levels are significantly higher [23, 24]. The differences in phosphate status between the two types of HF seems to be related to PTH, suggesting that PTH response to hypovitaminosis D is linked to an altered phosphate homeostasis [24]. Secondary hyperparathyroidism is a strong independent predictor of poor outcome in older patients, implying higher in-hospital mortality and higher rate of institutional care transfer after hospital discharge [27].

Hypovitaminosis D and Related Risk Factors in Patients with HF

Hypovitaminosis D as a Risk Factor for HF

The first studies analyzing the association between 25(OH)D levels and the risk of HF came from retrospective case-control studies and randomized clinical trials of vitamin D supplements. Results from these trials are quite contradictory, partly because the baseline 25(OH)D levels were not well known, since very often were only collected from a subgroup of participants, [57-61].

In case-control studies vitamin D status was measured at the time of fracture or shortly after it has occurred, and their results support a role for serum 25 (OH) D in fracture risk.

Some studies have prospectively analyzed the association between vitamin D status at recruitment and subsequent risk of fracture, with quite uniform results. The Study of Osteoporotic Fractures Research Group in the United States found, unlike other studies, that serum 25(OH)D levels were not associated with a subsequent risk of hip or vertebral fracture, but low levels of $1,25(OH)_2D$ were associated with a significant increased risk for HF [62].

The Malmo Osteoporosis prospective Risk Assessment (OPRA) study evaluated the association between 25(OH)D levels, fall-associated variables (physical activity, muscle strength) and fractures among ambulatory older Swedish women [63]. During the 3-year follow-up, 119 out of the 986 women sustained at least one fracture. The Cox proportional hazard ratio (HR) for suffering a fracture during the follow-up was 2.04 (95% CI: 1.04-4.04) for the group of women with 25(OH)D below 20 ng/ml. However a 25(OH)D level below 30 ng/ml was not associated with an increased risk of fractures in this study [HR: 1.01 (95% CI: 0.7-1.61)]. The two-fold increase in fracture risk in the subgroup of women with 25(OH)D levels below 20 ng/ml was associated with a lower physical activity and postural stability.

A report from the Third National Health and Nutrition Examination Survey (NHANES III, 1988-1994), used serum 25(OH)D data of 1,917 white men and women ≥65 years of age, and examined the relationship with incident HF risk [64]. They found 156 incident HF cases in the sample, and cases were older, had lower BMD, lower body mass index (BMI), more prevalent spine or wrist fractures, and consumed fewer kilocalories and less calcium. After adjusting for these differences, serum 25(OH)D levels were significantly related to HF. The multivariate-adjusted RR was 0.64 (95% CI, 0.46–0.89) among subjects with 25(OH)D levels >25 ng/ml compared to those with lower levels. When grouped into quartiles, the multivariate-adjusted RR for the second (20 ng/ml), third (25 ng/ml), and fourth (30 ng/ml) versus the first quartile (16 ng/ml) of serum 25(OH)D were 0.50 (95% CI, 0.25-1.00), 0.41 (95% CI, 0.24-0.70), and 0.50 (95% CI, 0.29-0.86), respectively, indicating that the relationship did not seem to be linear across all values.

Another prospective case-control study analyzed 400 cases of incident HF and 400 age and race-matched controls, with an average follow-up of 7.1 years [65]. The study population came from the Women's Health Initiative (WHI) Observational Study, a prospective cohort study that enrolled 93,676 community dwelling women aged 50–79 years from 1994–1998. The results showed that women with baseline 25(OH)D<19 ng/ml had an increased risk of subsequent HF over the next seven years, compared with women with 25(OH)D ≥28 ng/ml. In the WHI study for each 10 ng/ml decrease in 25(OH)D, the adjusted risk for fracture increased by 33% (OR= 1.33; 95% CI, 1.06-1.68) in multivariate models. Multivariate models included age, body mass index, parental and personal history of fractures, smoking, alcohol and calcium intake, geographic location and corticosteroid use. Women with the lowest 25(OH)D concentration (≤ 19 ng/ml) were at a higher risk of HF than women with the highest concentration (≥ 28 ng/ml). Compared with women with 25(OH)D ≥28 ng/ml, the OR of HF was 1.71 (95% CI, 1.05-2.79), 1.09 (95% CI, 0.70-1.71) and 0.82 (95% CI, 0.51-1.31) for women with 25(OH)D <19 ng/ml, 19-24 ng/ml and 24-28 ng/ml, respectively (p=0.015). The association between 25(OH)D and HF was observed in both women aged less than 70 and women aged 70 or older, and was independent of falls and frailty. These results suggest that measurement of 25(OH)D may be useful in identifying women at high risk of HF.

Result of the WHI study are consistent with the reports from NHANES III and OPRA studies, suggesting that serum 25(OH)D values exceeding 20-24 ng/ml are associated with lower risk of HF.

The association between vitamin D levels and incident fractures in older men has been less analyzed. With this objective a case-cohort study nested within the prospective Osteoporotic Fractures in Men Study was performed [66]. During the 5.3 years of follow-up, 435 incident non-vertebral fractures, including 81 HF, were observed in the entire cohort (5908 participants). The study sample for HF analysis was 1,665 men (1584 subcohort and 81 HF cases). Men who experienced a HF were older, had a lower BMI, lower vitamin D intake, lower mean 25(OH)D levels, lower BMD and worse neuromuscular function than men who did not experience a HF. The mean 25(OH)D levels were 16% lower in HF patients than in the subcohort, but interestingly there was no difference in total 25(OH)D levels between men with any nonvertebral fracture versus controls. Community-dwelling men with the lowest total 25(OH)D concentration (<19.9 ng/ml) at study entry had a greater than 2-fold increased risk of HF during the next 5 years compared with men with the highest total 25(OH)D level (≥27.9ng/ml)(HR = 2.36; 95% CI 1.08-5.16).

These HF results are consistent with the report from the NHANES III [64], that included 62 men with HF and 869 control men. Similar to the results of reports in older women, these findings suggest that low serum 25(OH)D concentrations may help to identify men at high risk of HF.

Risk Factors for Hypovitaminosis D

Several factors are associated with hypovitaminosis D development, such as advancing age, lack of physical activity, co-morbidities and frailty, low sun exposure, undernutrition or low functional status. Some of these factors often coincides in the same patient and specially in institutionalized patients.

Sun Exposure

There are few dietary sources of vitamin D, so the major source of vitamin D in humans is sunlight exposure [67, 68]. Factors that influence cutaneous vitamin D production include those depending on the patient (aging, skin pigmentation, sunscreen use) and those depending on the sun exposure (amount, time of day, season of the year and latitude). Several of these factors have shown to be associated with vitamin D deficiency in patients with HF. The degree of sun exposure during the previous three months is significantly associated with serum levels of 25(OH)D_3 in patients with HF [38]. The proportion of individuals with hypovitaminosis D was significantly lower in patients with greater sun exposure. In fact, an active sunlight exposure seems to be a protective factor for the presence of vitamin D deficiency (OR=0.09; 95% CI 0.02-0.5). A study conducted in 14 Mediterranean centres from Portugal, France, Italy, Spain, Greece and Turkey showed that lack of sunlight exposure in childhood, young adulthood or in the recent past is also an independent risk factor for HF in women over age 50 [69]. Although the habit of sunbathing is a modifiable factor and can increase the vitamin D status, we must take into account that in the latitudes in which Europe is located (Barcelona 41° N, Oslo 60° N), almost during winter months, the sun exposure does not allow the cutaneous photosynthesis of previtamin D [70].

Undernutrition

Undernutrition is a very common factor among elderly patients with HF [71, 72], mainly with intertrochanteric type [24]. Undernutrition is independently and strongly associated with hypovitaminosis D in patients with HF (OR=4.5; 95% IC 1.3-16.0) [38]. It is also important to highlight that vitamin D deficiency and undernutrition are often associated with other significant determinants of fracture risk, as renal dysfunction, in patients with HF [73, 74].

Functional Status

Functional status previous to hospital admission is another factor independently associated with hypovitaminosis D in patients with HF (OR=3; 95% IC 1.3-6.7) [38].

Serum 25(OH)D levels are also associated with the type of dwelling before admission, with higher prevalence of severe vitamin D deficiency in patients admitted from nursing homes [38, 48]. This is probably a reflection that these institutions agglutinate more disabled patients with poor nutrition and whose disability determines a higher indoor living with insufficient sunlight exposure.

Latitude

Evidence suggests a great heterogeneity in HF rate between countries, that may vary more than 10-fold between some of them [75, 76]. Maybe the main reason for these geographic variations is latitude. In fact, a significant association between 10-year HF risk and latitude has been demonstrated [77], For each increase in 10° of latitude, the risk of having a fracture increases by 0.6% (0.8 in women and 0.3% in men). This association between latitude and HF risk may be related to vitamin D status since the bioavailability of vitamin D largely depends on sunlight exposure, which decreases at higher latitudes.

Hypovitaminosis D and Other Risk Factors for Femoral Neck and Intertrochanteric HF

Vitamin D and Other Parameters of Bone Mineral Metabolism

Although no differences in vitamin D status have been found between individuals with intracapsular and extracapsular HF [23, 24], the type of fracture is significantly associated with PTH response to vitamin D deficiency and impaired phosphate homeostasis, as we have stated before [24]. In patients with either HF type (cervical or intertrochanteric), serum PTH, but not 25(OH)D, correlates positively with age, serum calcium and decline in renal function. Cervical HF patients show a significant inverse relationship between 25(OH)D and bone resorption markers, whereas in intertrochanteric HF patients 25(OH)D correlates negatively with bone formation markers (osteocalcin), and PTH correlates positively with serum bone-specific alkaline phosphatase and phosphate. The PTH response to hypovitaminosis D is a strong independent predictor of HF type (cervical vs intertrochanteric) in the multivariate analyses (OR=0.92; 95% CI 0.87-0.97). The coexistence of vitamin D deficiency and elevated PTH predicts intertrochanteric HF while coexistence of low vitamin D and non-elevated PTH was a strong predictor of cervical HF (OR= 3.50; 95% CI 1.52-7.98). In this publication each 1 pmol/L increase in serum PTH levels increased the risk of intertrochanteric vs. cervical HF about 10%. These results indicate that PTH response to vitamin D deficiency and the absolute level of PTH elevation may be major factors of bone and mineral metabolism contributing to HF type [24].

In patients with vitamin D deficiency with normal PTH, higher serum phosphate is a strong predictor of cervical vs trochanteric HF (RR=1.9; 95%CI 1.1-3.1). In contrast, in patients with vitamin D deficiency and secondary hyperparathyroidism higher phosphate levels are significantly associated with trochanteric fracture (RR=3.0; 95%CI 1.3-6.5) [24]. These results suggest that, in addition to the vitamin D–PTH axis, probably phosphate metabolism is strongly regulated by some other factors which act differently depending on the presence or absence of secondary hyperparathyroidism.

BMD and Geometrical Parameters

Low BMD is a well-established risk factor for HF [78] and the ability of BMD to discriminate cervical and intertrochanteric HF risk has been analyzed by different authors. A prospective study evaluated 192 HF (108 femoral neck and 84 intertrochanteric), occurring during an average follow-up of 4 years, among 5703 elderly women aged 75 years or more, who were recruited from the voting list in the EPIDOS study [79]. In women who sustained a HF, a significant decrease of femoral neck, trochanteric and whole body BMD bone measurements, was highly predictive of intertrochanteric fractures (RR= 3.2; CI 95% 2.4-4.2; RR=4.8; CI 95% 3.5-6.6; and RR=2.8; CI 95% 2.2-3.6, respectively) more accurately than cervical fractures (respectively, RR=2.1; CI 95% 1.7-2.7; RR=2.3; 1.8-3.0; and RR=1.2; 1.0-1.6). All ultrasound parameters, (SOS, BUA, and stiffness index) were significant predictors of intertrochanteric fractures (RR 3.0; CI 95% 2.2-4.1; RR 2.5; CI 95% 2.0-3.1; and RR 3.5; CI 95% 2.6-4.7, respectively) but not cervical fractures. Therefore, it seems that intertrochanteric fractures occur as a consequence of a generalized low BMD and calcaneal ultrasounds parameters, whereas other parameters could be involved in cervical fractures.

Many fractures occur among people not diagnosed as having osteoporosis (OP) based on the femoral neck BMD T-score. In a recent retrospective case-control study, the authors examined 57 postmenopausal females with HF and 40 controls, and investigated whether geometrical measures in femoral neck besides BMD can yield additional information for the assessment of HF risk [80]. Geometrical parameters (hip axis length, femoral neck axis length, femoral neck and shaft cortex thicknesses and femoral neck-shaft angle) were measured from digitized radiographs of the uninjured hip, and BMD was measured at the non-fracture side femoral neck and at left femoral neck in controls. The study suggested that the risk of intertrochanteric fracture could be discriminated based on a BMD T-score <-2.5 criterion, because only 5.6% of intertrochanteric fractures were classified as not having OP, whereas cervical fracture cases would remain under-diagnosed if solely this criterion was used (48.7% in the non-osteoporotic group). In fact, some geometrical parameters (wider neck-shaft angle and lesser cortical thickness at femoral neck) are able to discriminate cervical fracture cases, even among individuals with T-score >-2.5, though these findings need to be confirmed with a larger sample, preferably in a prospective study.

Risk Factors in Younger Patients

Knowledge about subjects who sustain a HF in middle age is poor. To investigate risk factors for HF occurring in this age group, Holmberg et al performed a sub-study with relevant data extracted from the Malmö Preventive Project [81]. This was a prospective, population-based, cardiovascular screening study started in the 1970s, with 22,444 men, and 10,902 women, mean age 50 years at inclusion. Follow up was up to 16 years with regard to occurrence of fracture. One hundred and thirty-five women had 135 HF (93 cervical and 42 intertrochanteric) and 163 men had 166 HF (81 cervical and 85 intertrochanteric). Many risk factors were similar for men and women, although the risk ratio differed. The risk factor pattern for cervical versus trochanteric fractures differed in both men and women, and only two risk factors were common to both fracture types in both sexes in the final Cox model: older age and low BMI. In women, a history of previous fractures was the strongest risk factor for cervical HF, with more than a 3-fold risk (RR=3.41; 95% CI 1.63-7.14) while for intertrochanteric HF a history of previous fractures and diabetes were very strong risk factors (RR=8.93; 95% CI 3.80-21.3 and RR=7.75; 95% CI 2.34-25.6, respectively). In men, the strongest risks factors for cervical HF were diabetes (RR=5.03; 95% CI 1.81-14.1) and current smoking (RR=2.09; 95% CI 1.25-3.47), while for trochanteric HF also diabetes and current smoking were the strongest risk factors (RR=8.81; 95% CI 3.77-20.4 and RR=2.42; 95% CI 1.44-4.07, respectively).

Some significant risk factors for trochanteric HF identified in this study were also risk factors for having low BMD. Since low BMD has been demonstrated in patients with trochanteric HF, the authors speculated that individuals suffering from trochanteric HF could also have low BMD already in middle age.

Seasonal Variation of HF Incidence

The seasonal incidence of HF has been shown in large population studies, conducted in very different geographical areas such as Taiwan [82], Spain [83], Hong Kong [84], United Kingdom [84, 85], New Zealand [84], Australia [86], Canada [87], Norway [88] or United States [89, 90]. In general, a higher incidence of fractures is observed in winter, a fact usually being associated with an increase in falls secondary to climatic conditions, like snow, rain and frost [86, 87, 89], but these variables do not seem to justify this seasonal presentation in certain geographical regions like our area, Barcelona (Spain), where snow and frost are both exceptional meteorological conditions. In addition, most of falls-related fractures occur indoor [89, 91, 92]. Other authors have demonstrated that this seasonal incidence of HF is closely associated with monthly temperature [82, 86], a finding not surprising since the peak for HF is during winter. As a general rule, the highest rate of fractures is observed in winter and the lowest in summer, although some series only show a decrease of cases during summer months [93]

As mentioned above, vitamin D deficiency is highly prevalent among elderly who have suffered an osteoporotic HF. On the other hand, it is also well known that vitamin D deficiency shows a seasonal variation, with winter predominance, in healthy elderly people [94, 95]. A recent study from our group has analyzed the possible relationship between this seasonal presentation of HF and vitamin D status of patients. Besides finding a significant lower incidence of HF in summer, we observed that patients who suffered the fracture during summer showed higher serum 25(OH)D3 levels and a trend to lower serum PTH levels compared to those who had HF in other seasons [93]. An observational, cross-sectional, population-based study set in Australia [latitude 38-39° S) with 1358 women studied the relationship between falls (1358 women presenting to hospital after falling), fractures (1635 women with incident fractures), serum 25(OH)D levels and PTH (287 women randomly selected from electoral rolls) and annual periodicities of ultraviolet radiation [96]. The authors reported annual periodicities in circulating 25(OH)D and PTH, with a decrease in 25(OH)D and an increase in PTH levels during winter, and a higher proportion of falls resulting in fracture, and a higher frequency of hip (and wrist) fractures. The cyclic variations in serum 25(OH)D lagged 1 month behind ultraviolet radiation, peaking in summer and dipping in winter ($p< 0.001$) and the periodicity of serum PTH was the inverse of serum 25(OH)D. In order to demonstrate the possible relationship between solar radiation, 25(OH)D3 levels and the incidence of seasonal osteoporotic HF, we evaluated a subgroup of patients with osteoporotic HF (Barcelona, 41°N) [97]. We excluded individuals without sun exposure (homebound or institutionalized), and those who had received vitamin D supplementation during the 6 months prior to the HF, because serum levels of 25(OH)D3 in those patients were not as related to the solar radiation. We observed an inverse correlation between the monthly number of fractures and 25(OH)D3 serum levels ($r=0.65$; $p=0.02$). In contrast, we observed a direct correlation between the 25(OH)D3 serum levels and the monthly average solar radiation for the 2nd and 3rd previous month ($r=0.69$; $p=0.013$ and $r=0.73$; $p=0.007$ respectively). Therefore the highest monthly solar radiation in our country is received around the summer solstice (late June), and the highest 25(OH)D3 levels are observed during the 2-3 following months, just in summer, when the incidence of HF is the lowest in our population.

A higher mortality among elderly patients hospitalized for HF has been reported during winter [84] which shows that patients are more fragile during this period. This circumstance could be related, at least in part, to a higher vitamin D deficiency during winter, and that these patients with lower vitamin D levels had a worse nutritional condition, a worse functional status, and more severe fractures [23, 38].

Importance of Hypovitaminosis D in the Clinical Presentation of HF

Myopathy

Vitamin D has some receptors in skeletal muscle [98] and play a role in muscle function, so in a situation of severe vitamin D deficiency, such as in osteomalacia, patients can develop a clinical myopathy [99]. Vitamin D deficiency has been shown to be associated with myopathy in subjects of different age [100-102] and with falls in institutionalized elderly subjects [103, 104]. It is well established that vitamin D deficiency increases postural instability through increased body sway and muscle weakness, and reduced ability to neutralize falls [102, 105, 106]. In a population-based cohort of Swedish elderly ambulatory women, the authors found that levels of 25(OH)D below 30 ng/ml were correlated with impaired balance, gait speed and physical activity compared with women above this threshold [63]. Some morphologic and histochemical changes in muscle fibres have been described in patients with HF. In a prospective, double-blind study some biopsies from the middle gluteus were performed at surgery in 42 elderly women with a HF due to a fall. The results of this investigation demonstrated that patients presented an atrophy of type II fibre in muscles that support the hip region. This atrophy correlates directly with the degree of vitamin D deficiency and was severe in patients with vitamin D deficiency. Patients with 25(OH)D levels <13 ng/ml had the type II fibre diameter significantly smaller than that in the sufficient group (25-OHD concentration >13 ng/ml). Furthermore, authors found that the mean type II fibre diameter correlated with serum 25(OH)D levels in the deficient group ($r = 0.714$, $p=0.0011$) [107]. Type II muscle fibres are the first to be recruited to prevent a fall, and some degree of atrophy of these fibres is common in the elderly [108]. Probably, both low physical activity and vitamin D deficiency may have caused the severe type II fibre atrophy in this deficient vitamin D group, and such morphologic changes may have weakened the support of the hip joint and lead to fall and HF in these patients.

Severity of Hip Fracture

*S*ome authors have evaluated whether risk factors for fracture could be different depending on severity of HF. A prospective study with older women followed up for over 10.5 years analyzed 462 first incident osteoporotic HF: 249 femoral neck fractures (30% undisplaced or grade I and II according to Garden Classification) (figure 3), and 213 intertrochanteric fractures (28% stable or grade I and II according to Kyle Classification) (figure 4) [109]. Older age was strongly associated with more severe fractures. Regarding femoral neck fractures, a 5-year increase in age was associated with an increased risk of undisplaced and displaced fractures (HR=1.70, 95% CI 1.40-2.06 and HR=1.81, 95% CI, 1.59-2.05, respectively) in age-adjusted models. Regarding intertrochanteric fractures, every 5-year increase in age was also associated with a increased risk of stable and unstable fractures (HR=2.10, 95% CI, 1.70-2.59 and HR=2.42, 95% CI, 2.14-2.75, respectively). We have also investigated the differences in baseline characteristics of patients with different severity types of osteoporotic HF and we found an association between vitamin D levels and HF severity [23]. We designed a cross-sectional study, including consecutive individuals over 65 years admitted to our hospital for osteoporotic HF during a year. Demographic data, fracture type, comorbidities, history of OP, functional and nutritional status, 25(OH)D3 and PTH levels were evaluated. In this series, 131 patients (40%) had less severe HF (femoral neck or intertrochanteric) and 193 patients (60%) more severe fractures. There was no difference in age and sex between groups. Individuals with more severe fractures showed significantly lower levels of 25OHD3 (20±15 ng/ml vs 26±21; p= 0.004) and higher prevalence of hypovitaminosis D (74% vs 57%; p = 0.002) compared with patients with less severe HF. Secondary hyperparathyroidism occurred more frequently among patients with more severe fractures (59% vs 48%; p=0.05) but no differences in other parameters were found between both groups. The multiple regression analysis confirmed the levels of 25OHD3 as the only independent variable associated with severe hip fracture (OR 0.98; 95% CI 0.97-0.99). In other words, for each 1ng/ml decrease in 25OHD3, the risk of having a severe HF increases about 2%. In our study, patients with hypovitaminosis D had a 47% higher risk of having a severe HF (OR 1.47; 95% CI 1.15-1.88). Our results can have some important clinical implications, highlighting a possible role of hypovitaminosis D in the severity of HF. This finding raises the hypothesis that a sufficient supplementation of vitamin D in patients at higher risk of HF could avoid the more severe types, those most closely associated with a poor functional outcome and higher mortality.

Concomitant Fractures

In a recent study, a group of women who sustained a HF and simultaneous fractures of the upper limb showed significantly lower levels of 25(OH)D than women without concomitant fractures (6.5±5.0 ng/ml vs 11.7±10.4 ng/ml respectively). This difference was also significant after adjustment for eight potential confounders, including age, height, weight, HF type, cognitive or neurological impairment, previous HF or upper-limb fractures, in this sample of older Italian women [110].

Vitamin D Treatment in HF

Primary Prevention

Supplementation with vitamin D and calcium is useful to lower the risk of HF, and most clinical guidelines for the prevention of HF recommend an intake of 800 IU vitamin D per day. Two meta-analysis concluded that a daily vitamin D oral supplementation between 700 to 800 IU of cholecalciferol, with or without calcium supplementation, reduced the risk of hip and any non-vertebral fractures in ambulatory or institutionalized elderly people [111, 112]. However, the use of additional calcium in all but one randomized controlled trials confounds interpretation of these meta-analysis. The critical question of whether vitamin D supplementation, either with or without calcium, is itself effective to prevent HF has been evaluated in a separate meta-analysis of randomised controlled trials and observational studies [113]. As a conclusion, neither higher nor lower doses of vitamin D supplementation were effective to prevent HF. As the authors comment, the reason for these results is unclear, and one possible explanation is uncontrolled confounding in observational studies.

In clinical practice, it is really alarming the low percentage of older patients on treatment for OP, many of them with risk factors that justify antiosteoporotic therapy which probably could have prevented HF in a great proportion of patients. In fact, only 4-20% of patients with HF was on vitamin D supplementation at admission in Europe or Australia [23, 24, 48] UK [47].

Secondary Prevention

Despite treatment with calcium and vitamin D has been shown effective to prevent new fractures after a HF, there is lack of diagnosis and treatment of OP after a HF, as well as an insufficient prescription of calcium and vitamin D supplements in these patients [114-119]. The strongest predictor of treatment with calcium and vitamin D after a HF is the prescription of antiresorptive or bone forming medication (OR=5.50, 95% CI: 4.84-6.25) [114]. Neither orthopaedic surgeons who treat HF nor primary physicians who provide long-term health care to the same patients appear to be engaged in secondary prevention.

Different studies of vitamin D supplementation in elderly HF patients have identified also problems of compliance with therapy [120-123], with about 25%-50% of patients being fully adherent to the supplement [121, 123]. Increasing age, presence of pain and no use of diagnostic test showed a positive effect on the probability of discontinuing the medication [121].

Supplementation with cholecalciferol (vitamin D3 metabolite) can be achieved equally well with daily, weekly, or monthly dosing frequencies. In fact, when cumulative dose and the vehicle of administration are the same, similar serum 25(OH)D concentrations are attained in older women with HF [124]. The supplementation with 1000 IU/day of cholecalciferol is more effective in increasing serum 25(OH)D than an equivalent dose of ergocalciferol (vitamin D2 metabolite) in vitamin D-insufficient HF patients [122].

Probably, vitamin D supplementation strategies using an easy posology with a wider interval of administration (weekly or monthly) could be more appropriate to optimize the individual adherence of these patients. We have previously reported the efficacy and safety of calcidiol (25(OH)D3 metabolite) to normalize and maintain vitamin D levels within the normal range. In a group of 129 rheumatology outpatients with hypovitaminosis D (25(OH)D3< 25 ng/ml) a simple regimen of 16,000 UI of calcidiol once weekly for 4 weeks was sufficient to normalize 25(OH)D3 levels [125], and 16,000 UI of calcidiol every 3 weeks were effective to maintain 25(OH)D3 levels within the normal range after a long-term treatment in nursing home residents with low vitamin D status [38]. A yearly administration of vitamin D can also be used, although it is not well established the safety of a high dose of vitamin D. A single year injection of 300,000 IU of vitamin D2 has been useful to reduce falls [120], but a single annual dose of 500.000 IU of cholecalciferol administered orally, resulted in an increased risk of falls and fractures [126].

The amelioration of the severity of OP (as measured by BMD) and the increase of serum 25(OH)D level after regular sunlight exposure have been demonstrated in stroke patients [127] and in elderly women with Alzheimer's disease [128] but not in patients with HF and low vitamin D levels.

Patients with a HF are at increased risk of fracturing the contralateral hip compared with subjects of similar age. About 10-12% of HF patients sustain a second HF [129, 130] in a mean interval of 3-5 years [129-131]. In a study carried out in Nottingham the incidence of the first fracture was 50 per 100.000 in women aged 55 to 64 years rising to 3760 in those aged 84 years and over. The incidence of a second fracture in younger women (55 to 64) years was 2344 per 100.000 whereas those over 84 years had a similar risk (2451 per 100 000) [132]. Treatment with calcium and vitamin D play an important role in the OP therapeutic strategy and in the prevention of HF. Despite this, there is little consensus over secondary prevention of HF. A small longitudinal observational study performed in elderly HF patients showed that after one year a significant lower rate of second HF was observed in patients treated with vitamin D and calcium supplements (with or without alendronate), with a RR of second HF 6-fold higher in the control group (RR=6.23; 95%CI 0.83-46.71) [133]. However, randomized studies evaluating the cost-efficacy of vitamin D (with or without calcium) in the reduction of a second HF as a primary end point are lacking.

Cholecalciferol supplementation in institutionalized and community-dwelling older individuals can reduce the overall rate of falls, as shown in several randomized trials and summarized in a meta-analysis [134], but the same therapy with 2000 IU/d after HF was not successful in reducing falls in a small randomized controlled trial [135]. In the same study this dose of cholecalciferol was successful in reducing by 55% the rate of hospital readmission during the 12-month follow-up and the rate of readmissions due to fall-related injury (60%) and infections (90%) [135]. Although these findings are based on a small number of individuals, it might have important clinical implications because clinical interventions in elderly HF patients are not well established.

Several studies have shown excess mortality among HF patients compared with the normal population of the same age. Therefore one of the endpoints of treatment should be to decrease mortality. In this sense, a prospective analysis evaluated if calcium and vitamin D supplementation is associated with survival in patients after HF [136]. The study population included 137 patients who were still alive after a median of 27.5 months after the fracture. The results of the study showed a 36% reduction in deaths in women, and 43% in men after 36 months of receiving calcium plus vitamin D supplementation. Survival of females who concomitantly used anti-osteoporotic drugs was higher, with a 43% reduction in mortality. However, this potential relationship between reduced mortality and post-fracture use of calcium and vitamin D supplementation needs to be verified in population-based, randomized, placebo-controlled trials with overall mortality as the main endpoint.

Conclusion

- The prevalence of hypovitaminosis D is high in patients with osteoporotic HF
- Measurement of 25(OH) D may be useful in identifying patients at high risk of HF
- 25(OH) D below 20 ng/ml increases the risk of HF
- Vitamin D deficiency is especially prevalent among HF patients with low sunlight exposure and low functional status
- HF has a seasonal incidence. There is an inverse correlation between the monthly number of fractures and 25(OH)D3 serum levels in HF patients
- Patients with vitamin D deficiency have more severe osteoporotic HF
- Vitamin D is a well tolerated and inexpensive prevention strategy for HF
- Current guidelines on vitamin D supplementation for the prevention of HF in older individuals are not sufficiently implemented.

References

[1] Eiskjaer S, Ostgard SE, Jakobsen BW, Jensen J, Lucht U. Years of potential life lost after hip fracture among postmenopausal women. *Acta. Orthop. Scand.* 1992; 63: 293-6.

[2] Knobel H, Diez A, Arnau D, Alier A, Ibanez J, Campodarve I, Supervia A, Nogues X. [The sequelae of osteoporotic femoral fracture in Barcelona]. *Med. Clin.* (Barc) 1992; 98: 441-4.

[3] Keene GS, Parker MJ, Pryor GA. Mortality and morbidity after hip fractures. *BMJ* 1993; 307: 1248-50.

[4] Sosa M, Segarra MC, Hernandez D, Gonzalez A, Liminana JM, Betancor P. Epidemiology of proximal femoral fracture in Gran Canaria (Canary Islands). *Age Ageing* 1993; 22: 285-8.

[5] Pages E, Cuxart A, Iborra J, Olona M, Bermejo B. [Factors associated with mortality and gait impairment in elderly patients with hip fractures]. *Med. Clin.* (Barc) 1998; 110: 687-91.

[6] Braithwaite RS, Col NF, Wong JB. Estimating hip fracture morbidity, mortality and costs. *J. Am. Geriatr. Soc.* 2003; 51: 364-70.

[7] Birge SJ, Morrow-Howell N, Proctor EK. Hip fracture. *Clin. Geriatr. Med.* 1994; 10: 589-609.

[8] De Laet RJ: Epidemiology of osteoporotic fractures in Europe. In: Marcus R FD, Kelsey J, editors., ed. Osteoporosis. San Diego: Academic, 2001; 585-97.

[9] Hernandez JL, Olmos JM, Alonso MA, Gonzalez-Fernandez CR, Martinez J, Pajaron M, Llorca J, Gonzalez-Macias J. Trend in hip fracture epidemiology over a 14-year period in a Spanish population. *Osteoporos Int.* 2006; 17: 464-70.

[10] Cooper C, Campion G, Melton LJ, 3rd. Hip fractures in the elderly: a world-wide projection. *Osteoporos Int.* 1992; 2: 285-9.

[11] Dhanwal DK, Dennison EM, Harvey NC, Cooper C. Epidemiology of hip fracture: Worldwide geographic variation. *Indian J. Orthop.* 2011; 45: 15-22.

[12] Icks A, Haastert B, Wildner M, Becker C, Meyer G. Trend of hip fracture incidence in Germany 1995-2004: a population-based study. *Osteoporos Int.* 2008; 19: 1139-45.

[13] Lawton JO, Baker MR, Dickson RA. Femoral neck fractures--two populations. *Lancet* 1983; 2: 70-2.

[14] Kenzora JE, McCarthy RE, Lowell JD, Sledge CB. Hip fracture mortality. Relation to age, treatment, preoperative illness, time of surgery, and complications. *Clin. Orthop. Relat. Res.* 1984: 45-56.

[15] Linton P. On the different types of fratures of the neck of the femur. *Acta Chir. Scand.* 1944; 90: 1-122.

[16] Ahlborg HG, Rosengren BE, Jarvinen TL, Rogmark C, Nilsson JA, Sernbo I, Karlsson MK. Prevalence of osteoporosis and incidence of hip fracture in women--secular trends over 30 years. *BMC Musculoskelet Disord*; 11: 48.

[17] Kannus P, Niemi S, Parkkari J, Palvanen M, Vuori I, Jarvinen M. Nationwide decline in incidence of hip fracture. *J. Bone Miner Res.* 2006; 21: 1836-8.

[18] Brauer CA, Coca-Perraillon M, Cutler DM, Rosen AB. Incidence and mortality of hip fractures in the United States. *Jama* 2009; 302: 1573-9.

[19] Garden R. Low-angle fixation in fractures of the femoral neck. *J. Bone Joint Surg. Br.* 1961: 647-664.

[20] Kyle RF, Gustilo RB, Premer RF. Analysis of six hundred and twenty-two intertrochanteric hip fractures. *J. Bone Joint Surg. Am.* 1979; 61: 216-21.

[21] Riggs BL, Wahner HW, Seeman E, Offord KP, Dunn WL, Mazess RB, Johnson KA, Melton LJ, 3rd. Changes in bone mineral density of the proximal femur and spine with aging. Differences between the postmenopausal and senile osteoporosis syndromes. *J. Clin. Invest.* 1982; 70: 716-23.

[22] Djuric M, Djonic D, Milovanovic P, Nikolic S, Marshall R, Marinkovic J, Hahn M. Region-specific sex-dependent pattern of age-related changes of proximal femoral cancellous bone and its implications on differential bone fragility. *Calcif Tissue Int.* 2010; 86: 192-201.

[23] Larrosa M, Gomez A, Casado E, Moreno M, Vazquez I, Orellana C, Berlanga E, Ramon J, Gratacos J. Hypovitaminosis D as a risk factor of hip fracture severity. *Osteoporos Int.* 2011.

[24] Fisher A, Srikusalanukul W, Davis M, Smith P. Hip fracture type: important role of parathyroid hormone (PTH) response to hypovitaminosis D. *Bone* 2010; 47: 400-7.

[25] Haentjens P, Autier P, Barette M, Venken K, Vanderschueren D, Boonen S. Survival and functional outcome according to hip fracture type: a one-year prospective cohort study in elderly women with an intertrochanteric or femoral neck fracture. *Bone* 2007; 41: 958-64.

[26] Aharonoff GB, Koval KJ, Skovron ML, Zuckerman JD. Hip fractures in the elderly: predictors of one year mortality. *J. Orthop. Trauma* 1997; 11: 162-5.

[27] Fisher A, Goh S, Srikusalanukul W, Davis M. Elevated serum PTH is independently associated with poor outcomes in older patients with hip fracture and vitamin D inadequacy. *Calcif. Tissue Int.* 2009; 85: 301-9.

[28] Karagiannis A, Papakitsou E, Dretakis K, Galanos A, Megas P, Lambiris E, Lyritis GP. Mortality rates of patients with a hip fracture in a southwestern district of Greece: ten-year follow-up with reference to the type of fracture. *Calcif. Tissue Int.* 2006; 78: 72-7.

[29] Jokinen H, Pulkkinen P, Korpelainen J, Heikkinen J, Keinanen-Kiukaanniemi S, Jamsa T, Korpelainen R. Risk factors for cervical and trochanteric hip fractures in elderly women: a population-based 10-year follow-up study. *Calcif. Tissue Int.* 2010; 87: 44-51.

[30] Greenspan SL, Myers ER, Maitland LA, Kido TH, Krasnow MB, Hayes WC. Trochanteric bone mineral density is associated with type of hip fracture in the elderly. *J. Bone Miner Res.* 1994; 9: 1889-94.

[31] Vega E, Mautalen C, Gomez H, Garrido A, Melo L, Sahores AO. Bone mineral density in patients with cervical and trochanteric fractures of the proximal femur. *Osteoporos Int.* 1991; 1: 81-6.

[32] Duboeuf F, Hans D, Schott AM, Kotzki PO, Favier F, Marcelli C, Meunier PJ, Delmas PD. Different morphometric and densitometric parameters predict cervical and trochanteric hip fracture: the EPIDOS Study. *J. Bone Miner Res.* 1997; 12: 1895-902.

[33] Stewart A, Porter RW, Primrose WR, Walker LG, Reid DM. Cervical and trochanteric hip fractures: bone mass and other parameters. *Clin. Rheumatol.* 1999; 18: 201-6.

[34] Bell KL, Loveridge N, Power J, Garrahan N, Meggitt BF, Reeve J. Regional differences in cortical porosity in the fractured femoral neck. *Bone* 1999; 24: 57-64.

[35] Partanen J, Jamsa T, Jalovaara P. Influence of the upper femur and pelvic geometry on the risk and type of hip fractures. *J. Bone Miner Res.* 2001; 16: 1540-6.

[36] Pulkkinen P, Eckstein F, Lochmuller EM, Kuhn V, Jamsa T. Association of geometric factors and failure load level with the distribution of cervical vs. trochanteric hip fractures. *J. Bone Miner Res.* 2006; 21: 895-901.

[37] Thomas MK, Lloyd-Jones DM, Thadhani RI, Shaw AC, Deraska DJ, Kitch BT, Vamvakas EC, Dick IM, Prince RL, Finkelstein JS. Hypovitaminosis D in medical inpatients. *N. Engl. J. Med.* 1998; 338: 777-83.

[38] Larrosa M, Gratacos J, Vaqueiro M, Prat M, Campos F, Roque M. [Prevalence of hypovitaminosis D in elderly institutionalized residents: influence of a substitutive treatment]. *Med. Clin.* (Barc) 2001; 117: 611-4.

[39] Mosekilde L. Vitamin D and the elderly. *Clin. Endocrinol.* (Oxf) 2005; 62: 265-81.

[40] Brown IR, Bakowska A, Millard PH. Vitamin D status of patients with femoral neck fractures. *Age Ageing* 1976; 5: 127-31.

[41] Baker MR, McDonnell H, Peacock M, Nordin BE. Plasma 25-hydroxy vitamin D concentrations in patients with fractures of the femoral neck. *Br. Med. J.* 1979; 1: 589.

[42] Lips P, Hackeng WH, Jongen MJ, van Ginkel FC, Netelenbos JC. Seasonal variation in serum concentrations of parathyroid hormone in elderly people. *J. Clin. Endocrinol. Metab.* 1983; 57: 204-6.

[43] von Knorring J, Slatis P, Weber TH, Helenius T. Serum levels of 25-hydroxyvitamin D, 24,25-dihydroxyvitamin D and parathyroid hormone in patients with femoral neck fracture in southern Finland. *Clin. Endocrinol.* (Oxf) 1982; 17: 189-94.

[44] Nurmi I, Kaukonen JP, Luthje P, Naboulsi H, Tanninen S, Kataja M, Kallio ML, Leppilampi M. Half of the patients with an acute hip fracture suffer from hypovitaminosis D: a prospective study in southeastern Finland. *Osteoporos Int.* 2005; 16: 2018-24.

[45] LeBoff MS, Kohlmeier L, Hurwitz S, Franklin J, Wright J, Glowacki J. Occult vitamin D deficiency in postmenopausal US women with acute hip fracture. *JAMA* 1999; 281: 1505-11.

[46] Sahota O, Gaynor K, Harwood RH, Hosking DJ. Hypovitaminosis D and 'functional hypoparathyroidism'-the NoNoF (Nottingham Neck of Femur) study. *Age Ageing* 2001; 30: 467-72.
[47] Moniz C, Dew T, Dixon T. Prevalence of vitamin D inadequacy in osteoporotic hip fracture patients in London. *Curr. Med. Res. Opin.* 2005; 21: 1891-4.
[48] Bischoff-Ferrari HA, Can U, Staehelin HB, Platz A, Henschkowski J, Michel BA, Dawson-Hughes B, Theiler R. Severe vitamin D deficiency in Swiss hip fracture patients. *Bone* 2008; 42: 597-602.
[49] Martinez ME, del Campo MT, Garcia JA, Sanchez-Cabezudo MJ, Medina S, Garc-ia Cimbrelo E, Munuera L. [Vitamin D levels in patients with hip fracture in Madrid]. *Med. Clin.* (Barc) 1996; 106: 41-4.
[50] Bakhtiyarova S, Lesnyak O, Kyznesova N, Blankenstein MA, Lips P. Vitamin D status among patients with hip fracture and elderly control subjects in Yekaterinburg, Russia. *Osteoporos Int.* 2006; 17: 441-6.
[51] Lal SK, Jacob KC, Nagi ON, Annamalai AL, Nair CR. Variations of some plasma components after closed fractures. *J. Trauma* 1976; 16: 206-11.
[52] Lips P, Bouillon R, Jongen MJ, van Ginkel FC, van der Vijgh WJ, Netelenbos JC. The effect of trauma on serum concentrations of vitamin D metabolites in patients with hip fracture. *Bone* 1985; 6: 63-7.
[53] Sahota O, Mundey MK, San P, Godber IM, Lawson N, Hosking DJ. The relationship between vitamin D and parathyroid hormone: calcium homeostasis, bone turnover, and bone mineral density in postmenopausal women with established osteoporosis. *Bone* 2004; 35: 312-9.
[54] Giusti A, Barone A, Razzano M, Pizzonia M, Oliveri M, Palummeri E, Pioli G. High prevalence of secondary hyperparathyroidism due to hypovitaminosis D in hospitalized elderly with and without hip fracture. *J. Endocrinol. Invest* 2006; 29: 809-13.
[55] DeLuca HF. 1,25-Dihydroxyvitamin D3 in the pathogenesis and treatment of osteoporosis. *Osteoporos Int.* 1997; 7 Suppl 3: S24-9.
[56] Lau EM, Woo J, Swaminathan R, MacDonald D, Donnan SP. Plasma 25-hydroxyvitamin D concentration in patients with hip fracture in Hong Kong. *Gerontology* 1989; 35: 198-204.
[57] Chapuy MC, Arlot ME, Delmas PD, Meunier PJ. Effect of calcium and cholecalciferol treatment for three years on hip fractures in elderly women. *BMJ* 1994; 308: 1081-2.
[58] Lips P, Graafmans WC, Ooms ME, Bezemer PD, Bouter LM. Vitamin D supplementation and fracture incidence in elderly persons. A randomized, placebo-controlled clinical trial. *Ann. Intern. Med.* 1996; 124: 400-6.
[59] Meyer HE, Smedshaug GB, Kvaavik E, Falch JA, Tverdal A, Pedersen JI. Can vitamin D supplementation reduce the risk of fracture in the elderly? A randomized controlled trial. *J. Bone Miner Res.* 2002; 17: 709-15.
[60] Chapuy MC, Pamphile R, Paris E, Kempf C, Schlichting M, Arnaud S, Garnero P, Meunier PJ. Combined calcium and vitamin D3 supplementation in elderly women: confirmation of reversal of secondary hyperparathyroidism and hip fracture risk: the Decalyos II study. *Osteoporos Int.* 2002; 13: 257-64.
[61] Trivedi DP, Doll R, Khaw KT. Effect of four monthly oral vitamin D3 (cholecalciferol) supplementation on fractures and mortality in men and women living in the community: randomised double blind controlled trial. *BMJ* 2003; 326: 469.

[62] Cummings SR, Browner WS, Bauer D, Stone K, Ensrud K, Jamal S, Ettinger B. Endogenous hormones and the risk of hip and vertebral fractures among older women. Study of Osteoporotic Fractures Research Group. *N. Engl. J. Med.* 1998; 339: 733-8.

[63] Gerdhem P, Ringsberg KA, Obrant KJ, Akesson K. Association between 25-hydroxy vitamin D levels, physical activity, muscle strength and fractures in the prospective population-based OPRA Study of Elderly Women. *Osteoporos Int.* 2005; 16: 1425-31.

[64] Looker AC, Mussolino ME. Serum 25-hydroxyvitamin D and hip fracture risk in older U.S. white adults. *J. Bone Miner Res.* 2008; 23: 143-50.

[65] Cauley JA, Lacroix AZ, Wu L, Horwitz M, Danielson ME, Bauer DC, Lee JS, Jackson RD, Robbins JA, Wu C, Stanczyk FZ, LeBoff MS, Wactawski-Wende J, Sarto G, Ockene J, Cummings SR. Serum 25-hydroxyvitamin D concentrations and risk for hip fractures. *Ann. Intern. Med.* 2008; 149: 242-50.

[66] Cauley JA, Parimi N, Ensrud KE, Bauer DC, Cawthon PM, Cummings SR, Hoffman AR, Shikany JM, Barrett-Connor E, Orwoll E. Serum 25-hydroxyvitamin D and the risk of hip and nonspine fractures in older men. *J. Bone Miner Res.* 2010; 25: 545-53.

[67] Holick MF. Resurrection of vitamin D deficiency and rickets. *J. Clin. Invest.* 2006; 116: 2062-72.

[68] Holick MF. Vitamin D deficiency. *N. Engl. J. Med.* 2007; 357: 266-81.

[69] Johnell O, Gullberg B, Kanis JA, Allander E, Elffors L, Dequeker J, Dilsen G, Gennari C, Lopes Vaz A, Lyritis G, et al. Risk factors for hip fracture in European women: the MEDOS Study. Mediterranean Osteoporosis Study. *J. Bone Miner Res.* 1995; 10: 1802-15.

[70] Webb AR, Kline L, Holick MF. Influence of season and latitude on the cutaneous synthesis of vitamin D3: exposure to winter sunlight in Boston and Edmonton will not promote vitamin D3 synthesis in human skin. *J. Clin. Endocrinol. Metab.* 1988; 67: 373-8.

[71] Patterson BM, Cornell CN, Carbone B, Levine B, Chapman D. Protein depletion and metabolic stress in elderly patients who have a fracture of the hip. *J. Bone Joint Surg. Am.* 1992; 74: 251-60.

[72] Jensen JE, Jensen TG, Smith TK, Johnston DA, Dudrick SJ. Nutrition in orthopaedic surgery. *J. Bone Joint Surg. Am.* 1982; 64: 1263-72.

[73] Ensrud KE, Lui LY, Taylor BC, Ishani A, Shlipak MG, Stone KL, Cauley JA, Jamal SA, Antoniucci DM, Cummings SR. Renal function and risk of hip and vertebral fractures in older women. *Arch. Intern. Med.* 2007; 167: 133-9.

[74] LaCroix AZ, Lee JS, Wu L, Cauley JA, Shlipak MG, Ott SM, Robbins J, Curb JD, Leboff M, Bauer DC, Jackson RD, Kooperberg CL, Cummings SR. Cystatin-C, renal function, and incidence of hip fracture in postmenopausal women. *J. Am. Geriatr. Soc.* 2008; 56: 1434-41.

[75] Bacon WE, Maggi S, Looker A, Harris T, Nair CR, Giaconi J, Honkanen R, Ho SC, Peffers KA, Torring O, Gass R, Gonzalez N. International comparison of hip fracture rates in 1988-89. *Osteoporos Int.* 1996; 6: 69-75.

[76] Elffors I, Allander E, Kanis JA, Gullberg B, Johnell O, Dequeker J, Dilsen G, Gennari C, Lopes Vaz AA, Lyritis G, et al. The variable incidence of hip fracture in southern Europe: the MEDOS Study. *Osteoporos Int.* 1994; 4: 253-63.

[77] Johnell O, Borgstrom F, Jonsson B, Kanis J. Latitude, socioeconomic prosperity, mobile phones and hip fracture risk. *Osteoporos Int.* 2007; 18: 333-7.

[78] Bruyere O, Varela AR, Adami S, Detilleux J, Rabenda V, Hiligsmann M, Reginster JY. Loss of hip bone mineral density over time is associated with spine and hip fracture incidence in osteoporotic postmenopausal women. *Eur. J. Epidemiol.* 2009; 24: 707-12.

[79] Schott AM, Hans D, Duboeuf F, Dargent-Molina P, Hajri T, Breart G, Meunier PJ. Quantitative ultrasound parameters as well as bone mineral density are better predictors of trochanteric than cervical hip fractures in elderly women. Results from the EPIDOS study. *Bone* 2005; 37: 858-63.

[80] Pulkkinen P, Partanen J, Jalovaara P, Jamsa T. BMD T-score discriminates trochanteric fractures from unfractured controls, whereas geometry discriminates cervical fracture cases from unfractured controls of similar BMD. *Osteoporos Int.* 2010; 21: 1269-76.

[81] Holmberg AH, Johnell O, Nilsson PM, Nilsson JA, Berglund G, Akesson K. Risk factors for hip fractures in a middle-aged population: a study of 33,000 men and women. *Osteoporos Int.* 2005; 16: 2185-94.

[82] Lin HC, Xiraxagar S. Seasonality of hip fractures and estimates of season-attributable effects: a multivariate ARIMA analysis of population-based data. *Osteoporos Int.* 2006; 17: 795-806.

[83] Alvarez-Nebreda ML, Jimenez AB, Rodriguez P, Serra JA. Epidemiology of hip fracture in the elderly in Spain. *Bone* 2008; 42: 278-85.

[84] Douglas S, Bunyan A, Chiu KH, Twaddle B, Maffulli N. Seasonal variation of hip fracture at three latitudes. *Injury* 2000; 31: 11-9.

[85] Crawford JR, Parker MJ. Seasonal variation of proximal femoral fractures in the United Kingdom. *Injury* 2003; 34: 223-5.

[86] Lau EM, Gillespie BG, Valenti L, O'Connell D. The seasonality of hip fracture and its relationship with weather conditions in New South Wales. *Aust. J. Public Health* 1995; 19: 76-80.

[87] Levy AR, Bensimon DR, Mayo NE, Leighton HG. Inclement weather and the risk of hip fracture. *Epidemiology* 1998; 9: 172-7.

[88] Gronskag AB, Forsmo S, Romundstad P, Langhammer A, Schei B. Incidence and seasonal variation in hip fracture incidence among elderly women in Norway. The HUNT Study. *Bone* 2010; 46: 1294-8.

[89] Mirchandani S, Aharonoff GB, Hiebert R, Capla EL, Zuckerman JD, Koval KJ. The effects of weather and seasonality on hip fracture incidence in older adults. *Orthopedics* 2005; 28: 149-55.

[90] Bischoff-Ferrari HA, Orav JE, Barrett JA, Baron JA. Effect of seasonality and weather on fracture risk in individuals 65 years and older. *Osteoporos Int.* 2007; 18: 1225-33.

[91] Aharonoff GB, Dennis MG, Elshinawy A, Zuckerman JD, Koval KJ. Circumstances of falls causing hip fractures in the elderly. *Clin. Orthop. Relat. Res.* 1998: 10-4.

[92] Sanders KM, Seeman E, Ugoni AM, Pasco JA, Martin TJ, Skoric B, Nicholson GC, Kotowicz MA. Age- and gender-specific rate of fractures in Australia: a population-based study. *Osteoporos Int.* 1999; 10: 240-7.

[93] Larrosa M GA, Gratacós J, Casado E, Fernández E, Berlanga E. Seasonal presentation of osteoporotic hip fracture: relation to 25(OH)D3 levels. *Ann. Rheum. Dis.* 2004; 63: 460-1.

[94] Hegarty V, Woodhouse P, Khaw KT. Seasonal variation in 25-hydroxyvitamin D and parathyroid hormone concentrations in healthy elderly people. *Age Ageing* 1994; 23: 478-82.

[95] Melin A, Wilske J, Ringertz H, Saaf M. Seasonal variations in serum levels of 25-hydroxyvitamin D and parathyroid hormone but no detectable change in femoral neck bone density in an older population with regular outdoor exposure. *J. Am. Geriatr. Soc.* 2001; 49: 1190-6.
[96] Pasco JA, Henry MJ, Kotowicz MA, Sanders KM, Seeman E, Pasco JR, Schneider HG, Nicholson GC. Seasonal periodicity of serum vitamin D and parathyroid hormone, bone resorption, and fractures: the Geelong Osteoporosis Study. *J. Bone Miner Res.* 2004; 19: 752-8.
[97] Larrosa M GA, Gratacós J, Casado E, Fernández E, Berlanga E. Sunlight irradiation, 25(OH)D3 serum levels and osteoporotic hip fracture. *Ann. Rheum. Dis.* 2004; 63: 462-3.
[98] Simpson RU, Thomas GA, Arnold AJ. Identification of 1,25-dihydroxyvitamin D3 receptors and activities in muscle. *J. Biol. Chem.* 1985; 260: 8882-91.
[99] Skaria J, Katiyar BC, Srivastava TP, Dube B. Myopathy and neuropathy associated with osteomalacia. *Acta Neurol. Scand.* 1975; 51: 37-58.
[100] Bischoff HA, Stahelin HB, Urscheler N, Ehrsam R, Vonthein R, Perrig-Chiello P, Tyndall A, Theiler R. Muscle strength in the elderly: its relation to vitamin D metabolites. *Arch. Phys. Med. Rehabil.* 1999; 80: 54-8.
[101] Mowe M, Haug E, Bohmer T. Low serum calcidiol concentration in older adults with reduced muscular function. *J. Am. Geriatr. Soc.* 1999; 47: 220-6.
[102] Glerup H, Mikkelsen K, Poulsen L, Hass E, Overbeck S, Andersen H, Charles P, Eriksen EF. Hypovitaminosis D myopathy without biochemical signs of osteomalacic bone involvement. *Calcif. Tissue Int.* 2000; 66: 419-24.
[103] Bischoff HA, Stahelin HB, Dick W, Akos R, Knecht M, Salis C, Nebiker M, Theiler R, Pfeifer M, Begerow B, Lew RA, Conzelmann M. Effects of vitamin D and calcium supplementation on falls: a randomized controlled trial. *J. Bone Miner Res.* 2003; 18: 343-51.
[104] Stein MS, Wark JD, Scherer SC, Walton SL, Chick P, Di Carlantonio M, Zajac JD, Flicker L. Falls relate to vitamin D and parathyroid hormone in an Australian nursing home and hostel. *J. Am. Geriatr. Soc.* 1999; 47: 1195-201.
[105] Pfeifer M, Begerow B, Minne HW, Abrams C, Nachtigall D, Hansen C. Effects of a short-term vitamin D and calcium supplementation on body sway and secondary hyperparathyroidism in elderly women. *J. Bone Miner Res.* 2000; 15: 1113-8.
[106] Gloth FM, 3rd, Smith CE, Hollis BW, Tobin JD. Functional improvement with vitamin D replenishment in a cohort of frail, vitamin D-deficient older people. *J. Am. Geriatr. Soc.* 1995; 43: 1269-71.
[107] Sato Y, Inose M, Higuchi I, Higuchi F, Kondo I. Changes in the supporting muscles of the fractured hip in elderly women. *Bone* 2002; 30: 325-30.
[108] Lexell J, Taylor CC, Sjostrom M. What is the cause of the ageing atrophy? Total number, size and proportion of different fiber types studied in whole vastus lateralis muscle from 15- to 83-year-old men. *J. Neurol. Sci.* 1988; 84: 275-94.
[109] Cauley JA, Lui LY, Genant HK, Salamone L, Browner W, Fink HA, Cohen P, Hillier T, Bauer DC, Cummings SR. Risk factors for severity and type of the hip fracture. *J. Bone Miner Res.* 2009; 24: 943-55.
[110] Di Monaco M, Vallero F, Castiglioni C, Di Monaco R, Tappero R. Low levels of 25-hydroxyvitamin D are associated with the occurrence of concomitant upper limb

fractures in older women who sustain a fall-related fracture of the hip. *Maturitas* 2011; 68: 79-82.

[111] Bischoff-Ferrari HA, Willett WC, Wong JB, Giovannucci E, Dietrich T, Dawson-Hughes B. Fracture prevention with vitamin D supplementation: a meta-analysis of randomized controlled trials. *JAMA* 2005; 293: 2257-64.

[112] Bischoff-Ferrari HA, Willett WC, Wong JB, Stuck AE, Staehelin HB, Orav EJ, Thoma A, Kiel DP, Henschkowski J. Prevention of nonvertebral fractures with oral vitamin D and dose dependency: a meta-analysis of randomized controlled trials. *Arch. Intern. Med.* 2009; 169: 551-61.

[113] Lai JK, Lucas RM, Clements MS, Roddam AW, Banks E. Hip fracture risk in relation to vitamin D supplementation and serum 25-hydroxyvitamin D levels: a systematic review and meta-analysis of randomised controlled trials and observational studies. *BMC Public Health* 2010; 10: 331.

[114] Jennings LA, Auerbach AD, Maselli J, Pekow PS, Lindenauer PK, Lee SJ. Missed opportunities for osteoporosis treatment in patients hospitalized for hip fracture. *J. Am. Geriatr. Soc.* 2010; 58: 650-7.

[115] Harrington JT, Broy SB, Derosa AM, Licata AA, Shewmon DA. Hip fracture patients are not treated for osteoporosis: a call to action. *Arthritis Rheum* 2002; 47: 651-4.

[116] Petrella RJ, Jones TJ. Do patients receive recommended treatment of osteoporosis following hip fracture in primary care? *BMC Fam. Pract.* 2006; 7: 31.

[117] Luthje P, Nurmi-Luthje I, Kaukonen JP, Kuurne S, Naboulsi H, Kataja M. Undertreatment of osteoporosis following hip fracture in the elderly. *Arch. Gerontol. Geriatr.* 2009; 49: 153-7.

[118] Follin SL, Black JN, McDermott MT. Lack of diagnosis and treatment of osteoporosis in men and women after hip fracture. *Pharmacotherapy* 2003; 23: 190-8.

[119] Fisher AA, Davis MW, Smith PN. Undertreatment of osteoporosis following hip fracture. *J. Bone Joint Surg. Am.* 2003; 85-A: 1394-5; author reply 1395-6.

[120] Harwood RH, Sahota O, Gaynor K, Masud T, Hosking DJ. A randomised, controlled comparison of different calcium and vitamin D supplementation regimens in elderly women after hip fracture: The Nottingham Neck of Femur (NONOF) Study. *Age Ageing* 2004; 33: 45-51.

[121] Carnevale V, Nieddu L, Romagnoli E, Bona E, Piemonte S, Scillitani A, Minisola S. Osteoporosis intervention in ambulatory patients with previous hip fracture: a multicentric, nationwide Italian survey. *Osteoporos Int.* 2006; 17: 478-83.

[122] Glendenning P, Chew GT, Seymour HM, Gillett MJ, Goldswain PR, Inderjeeth CA, Vasikaran SD, Taranto M, Musk AA, Fraser WD. Serum 25-hydroxyvitamin D levels in vitamin D-insufficient hip fracture patients after supplementation with ergocalciferol and cholecalciferol. *Bone* 2009; 45: 870-5.

[123] Segal E, Zinman C, Raz B, Ish-Shalom S. Low patient compliance--a major negative factor in achieving vitamin D adequacy in elderly hip fracture patients supplemented with 800IU of vitamin D3 daily. *Arch. Gerontol. Geriatr.* 2009; 49: 364-7.

[124] Ish-Shalom S, Segal E, Salganik T, Raz B, Bromberg IL, Vieth R. Comparison of daily, weekly, and monthly vitamin D3 in ethanol dosing protocols for two months in elderly hip fracture patients. *J. Clin. Endocrinol. Metab.* 2008; 93: 3430-5.

[125] Larrosa M, Casado E, Vazquez I, Navarro N, Gratacos J. Comment on Przybelski et al.: Rapid correction of low vitamin D status in nursing home residents. *Osteoporos Int.* 2009; 20: 1455-6.
[126] Sanders KM, Stuart AL, Williamson EJ, Simpson JA, Kotowicz MA, Young D, Nicholson GC. Annual high-dose oral vitamin D and falls and fractures in older women: a randomized controlled trial. *JAMA* 2010; 303: 1815-22.
[127] Sato Y, Metoki N, Iwamoto J, Satoh K. Amelioration of osteoporosis and hypovitaminosis D by sunlight exposure in stroke patients. *Neurology* 2003; 61: 338-42.
[128] Sato Y, Iwamoto J, Kanoko T, Satoh K. Amelioration of osteoporosis and hypovitaminosis D by sunlight exposure in hospitalized, elderly women with Alzheimer's disease: a randomized controlled trial. *J. Bone Miner Res.* 2005; 20: 1327-33.
[129] Kaukonen JP, Luthje P, Nurmi-Luthje I, Kataja M, Naboulsi H. Second hip fracture and patients' medication after the first hip fracture: a follow-up of 221 hip fracture patients in Finland. *Arch. Gerontol. Geriatr.* 2011; 52: 185-9.
[130] Gaumetou E, Zilber S, Hernigou P. Non-simultaneous bilateral hip fracture: Epidemiologic study of 241 hip fractures. *Orthop. Traumatol. Surg. Res.* 2011; 97: 22-7.
[131] Schroder HM, Petersen KK, Erlandsen M. Occurrence and incidence of the second hip fracture. *Clin. Orthop. Relat. Res.* 1993: 166-9.
[132] Lawrence TM, Wenn R, Boulton CT, Moran CG. Age-specific incidence of first and second fractures of the hip. *J. Bone Joint Surg. Br.* 2010; 92: 258-61.
[133] Segal E, Zinnman C, Raz B, Tamir A, Gurevich B, Siebzehner MI, Ish-Shalom S. Second hip fracture in elderly hip fracture patients: cost and effectiveness of fracture prevention treatment. *Age Ageing* 2005; 34: 507-10.
[134] Bischoff-Ferrari HA, Dawson-Hughes B, Staehelin HB, Orav JE, Stuck AE, Theiler R, Wong JB, Egli A, Kiel DP, Henschkowski J. Fall prevention with supplemental and active forms of vitamin D: a meta-analysis of randomised controlled trials. *BMJ* 2009; 339: b3692.
[135] Bischoff-Ferrari HA, Dawson-Hughes B, Platz A, Orav EJ, Stahelin HB, Willett WC, Can U, Egli A, Mueller NJ, Looser S, Bretscher B, Minder E, Vergopoulos A, Theiler R. Effect of high-dosage cholecalciferol and extended physiotherapy on complications after hip fracture: a randomized controlled trial. *Arch. Intern. Med.* 2010; 170: 813-20.
[136] Nurmi-Luthje I, Luthje P, Kaukonen JP, Kataja M, Kuurne S, Naboulsi H, Karjalainen K. Post-fracture prescribed calcium and vitamin D supplements alone or, in females, with concomitant anti-osteoporotic drugs is associated with lower mortality in elderly hip fracture patients: a prospective analysis. *Drugs Aging* 2009; 26: 409-21.

In: Vitamin D Deficiency
Editors: V. Lerner and C. Miodownik
ISBN: 978-1-61470-964-0

Chapter VI

Vitamin D, Nutritional Imprinting and Prostate Cancer

Jovana Kaludjerovic*[*1], Dennis Wagner[1,2], Wendy E. Ward[3] and Reinhold Vieth[1,2]

[1] Department of Nutritional Sciences, Faculty of Medicine, University of Toronto, Canada

[2] Department of Pathology and Laboratory Medicine, University of Toronto and Mount Sinai Hospital, Canada

[3] Department of Kinesiology, Centre for Bone and Muscle Health, Faculty of Applied Health Sciences, Brock University, Canada

Abstract

The fetal-origin hypothesis has reshaped the way of scientific thinking by identifying that the in utero and postnatal metabolic environment can be memorized by the developing organism through fetal and neonatal imprinting. In light of this hypothesis, prenatal and postnatal events can be thought of as the foundation for structural and functional development of an organism. An example of such a prenatal event includes a nutritional inadequacy that may have long-term consequences for health.

For example, vitamin D inadequacy during prenatal and early neonatal life has been associated with an increased risk for nutritional rickets, failure to thrive, osteomalacia and osteoporosis. Emerging evidence also suggests that long-term vitamin D inadequacy is implicated in many chronic diseases including cancer. This chapter discusses the role of vitamin D in nutritional imprinting and, specifically, the potential effect of vitamin D in modulating risk of prostate cancer.

[*] Correspondence author: Jovana Kaludjerovic, M.Sc. Department of Nutritional Sciences, Faculty of Medicine, University of Toronto, FitzGerald Bldg, 150 College St., Toronto, Ontario, Canada M5S 3E2. Phone: 647-292-5639; Fax: 416-978-5882; E-mail: jovana.kaludjerovic@utoronto.ca.

Abbreviations

1α-OHase	1α-hydroxylase;
$1,25(OH)_2D$	1,25-dihydroxyvitamin D;
24-OHase	24-hydroxylase;
25-OHase	25-hydroxylase;
25(OH)D	25-hydroxyvitamin D;
AIPCa	androgen-independent prostate cancer;
AR	androgen receptor;
ASCENT	AIPCa Study of Calcitriol Enhancing Taxotere;
$CaBP_{28K}$	calbindin-D_{28K};
IGF-1	insulin-like growth factor-1;
IL	interleukin;
IU	international unit;
NHANES	National Health and Nutrition Examination Survey;
PCa	prostate cancer;
PSA	prostate specific antigen;
PTH	parathyroid hormone;
RDA	ecommended dietary allowance;
TNF-α/ß	tumor necrosis factor-α/ß;
VDBP	vitamin D binding protein;
VDR	vitamin D receptor;
VDRE	vitamin D response element;
UV-B	ultraviolet-B.

Nutritional Imprinting

In 1974, Professor Günter Dörner suggested that the concentration of hormones, metabolites, and neurotransmitters present in early life can program brain development and function, as well as syndromes of reproduction and metabolism in human adults [1, 2]. He also proposed that during development there is an interaction between an individual's genetic makeup and the environment which determines later function in adult life [2]. In 1989, this concept was confirmed by Dr. David Barker when he showed, using data from cohorts of individuals born in the first half of the 20th century, that infants with lower body weight at birth and at one year of age have a higher risk of coronary heart disease, hypertension and stroke in adulthood [3]. This research led Barker and colleagues to develop the fetal-origin hypothesis. The fetal-origin hypothesis stipulates that prenatal and neonatal exposures, such as nutritional inadequacy, are memorized by the developing organism through the process of fetal and neonatal imprinting [4]. In light of this hypothesis, early life nutrition can be thought of as the foundation for structural and functional development of an organism.

During development, the fetus is nourished (via the placenta) through diet and mobilization of maternal nutrient stores. Thus, maternal nutrition before and during gestation is thought to be the single most important environmental factor influencing fetal development and pregnancy outcomes. Mothers who have adequate nutrient stores prior to pregnancy and consume a balanced diet during gestation are able to provide well for their offspring. Mothers who have an inadequate supply of nutrients, vitamins or minerals have to compete with their offspring for the available food supply. This competition limits the amount of nutrients delivered to the fetus and can have serious consequences on the well-being of both organisms. Emerging evidence indicates that an undernourished fetus may adapt to expand the surface area of its placenta to extract more nutrients from the mother [5]. Although this adaptation is needed to increase the survival of the fetus, it has adverse effects on fetal growth and development. Godfrey et al. [6] showed that placental size is inversely associated with the risk of metabolic disease in adulthood. This may be because a larger placenta requires a greater portion of nutrients, leaving the fetus in a nutritionally scarce environment. Under these conditions, the fetus uses an adaptive response and diverts the available nutrients and oxygenated blood away from body organs to spare brain development and function [7, 8]. This limits the growth of many fetal organs including the liver, which regulates cholesterol as well as vitamin D metabolism. Barker et al. [8, 9] showed that men who had smaller body size in relation to head size at birth had persisting disturbances in cholesterol metabolism, blood coagulation and higher rates of coronary heart disease at adulthood. To our knowledge, no studies have explored how restrictions in fetal liver growth affect vitamin D metabolism and function. It has also been hypothesized that an undernourished fetus receives signals that nutritional availability is scarce in the postnatal environment. These signals are believed to trigger metabolic adaptations in the developing fetus that reduce its energy demands and alter its epigenetic programming [10]. Thus, the process that underlies differential risk of disease is in part mediated by differences in nutrient availability during development; however, the role of individual nutrients is not well understood. Evidence is accumulating that vitamin D is a critical modulator of human health, and that vitamin D inadequacy can modify developmental trajectory and predispose the individual to lifelong health problems including most metabolic diseases and several types of malignancies [11].

Vitamin D Intake

Vitamin D_3 (cholecalciferol) is produced naturally in skin exposed to ultraviolet B (UV-B) sunlight. As a result, a common misconception is that 20-30 min of daily sunlight exposure precludes the need to consume vitamin D supplements. However, only prehistoric humans who inhabited tropical Africa and exposed their full body surface to daily sunlight could meet their vitamin D needs from sunlight exposure [12]. In contrast, modern humans who typically cover 95% of their body with clothing, wear sunscreen, and spend much of their time indoors do not produce sufficient levels of vitamin D from sun exposure [12]. According to some predictions, the average vitamin D supply of prehistoric humans was likely more than 10,000 International Units (IU)/d [13], while that of modern humans is substantially lower (approximately 400 IU/d) [12]. There are many variables that limit the photosynthesis and bioavailability of vitamin D. Some of these factors include limited sun exposure due to latitude, season, time of day, atmospheric components, clothing and sunscreen use, as well as skin pigmentation, age, obesity and certain diseases [14]. Thus, oral consumption of vitamin D is required in the current environment to achieve adequate vitamin D nutrition (Table 1).

Table 1. Classification of vitamin D replete and deficient states by serum 25(OH)D levels[a, b]

Classification	Serum 25(OH)D (nmol/L)	Outcomes
Deficient	≤25	High bone turnover High risk of osteomalacia and rickets [150]
Insufficient	27.5-50	Increased bone turnover Increased risk of osteomalacia and bone disorders Inadequate for bone and overall health [150]
Replete	>50	Adequate for bone health [150]
Optimal	>75	Suggested as a desirable concentration for overall health and disease prevention [24, 30, 151]
Toxic	>375	Pose a risk of adverse effects and have a potential for toxicity [151]

[a] 25(OH)D = 25-hydroxyvitamin D.
[b] To convert from nmol/L to ng/mL, divide by 2.496.

The major dietary sources of vitamin D include fish (e.g. salmon, tuna and mackerel) and fish liver oils with smaller amounts of vitamin D present in beef, egg yolk and some forms of mushrooms [15]. According to the 2005-2006 National Health and Nutrition Examination Survey (NHANES), average vitamin D intake levels in the United States range from 204-288 IU/d for males and 144-276 IU/d for females [16]. When vitamin D supplements were included in the analyses mean vitamin D intakes increased by 400 IU/d as this was the Recommended Dietary Allowance (RDA) for vitamin D at the time the survey was conducted [17]. Currently, there is no available data for vitamin D intake for infants 0 to 12 months or for pregnant and lactating women because the surveyed sample size for these population groups was too small to provide nationally representative estimates [16]. Given the physiological importance of vitamin D and its limited availability from sunlight exposure and diet, supplementation with vitamin D is often required. This need becomes even more significant during sensitive stages of development, including the prenatal and neonatal stages of life [18]. As of November 2010, the RDA for vitamin D in North America is 600 IU/d for men and women (1 to 70 years of age) and 800 IU/d for older adults [17]. The RDA for pregnant and/or lactating women is the same as for men and women from 1-70 years of age. According to the Institute of Medicine's Food and Nutrition Board there is no evidence that pregnant and/or lactating women require more vitamin D or serum 25(OH)D than non-pregnant women, or that maternal 25(OH)D levels modulate fetal calcium homeostasis. This conclusion is based on findings from one randomized control trial published in 1986, and 14 observational studies. A pilot trial published in 2008, showed that maternal vitamin D supplementation of 6400 IU/d for 6 months can ensure that both the mother and the infant have adequate 25(OH)D status (>50 nmol/L), and that their serum and urinary calcium are in the normal range [19]. To date, the Canadian Paediatric Society has made a recommendation for higher doses of vitamin D (2000 IU daily) to be taken by women during pregnancy [20].

Vitamin D Physiology

Vitamin D, derived from the skin or consumed orally, undergoes two hydroxylation steps in the body [21]. First, the vitamin D binding protein (VDBP) transports the inactive vitamin D molecule to the liver where it is hydroxylated by the 25-hydroxylase enzyme (25-OHase; CYP27A1) to form 25-hydroxyvitamin D [25(OH)D], the main circulating vitamin D metabolite and the clinical measure of vitamin D status in routine laboratory testing [21, 22]. Next, 1α-hydroxylase (1α-OHase; CYP27B1) in the kidney converts 25(OH)D into 1,25-dihydroxyvitamin D (1,25$(OH)_2$D), the biologically active hormone. Renal 24-hydroxylase (24-OHase; CYP24A1) catalyzes the catabolism of vitamin D metabolites into water-soluble breakdown products (i.e. calcitroic acid) that are ultimately excreted in the urine or bile [21].

The classical endocrine function of 1,25$(OH)_2$D is to maintain blood calcium homeostasis and optimize bone health by increasing the efficiency of dietary calcium absorption from the small intestine. Renal production of 1,25$(OH)_2$D is tightly regulated by negative feedback, as well as serum calcium, phosphorus, or parathyroid hormone (PTH) [23]. Under conditions of inadequate dietary calcium, 1,25$(OH)_2$D works in conjunction with PTH to mobilize calcium from bone by activating osteoclasts. The beneficial effects of vitamin D ($\geq$ 800 IU/d) on skeletal health include enhanced calcium absorption, suppression of PTH, improved muscle function (i.e. less falls) and reduced risk of osteoporotic hip fractures [24, 25].

Many non-renal tissues (i.e. heart, brain, skin, colon, breast, prostate, skeletal muscle, nerves, placenta and several others) also express 1α-OHase and therefore have the capacity to locally convert 25(OH) D to 1,25$(OH)_2$D [26, 27]. Several of these extra-renal tissues also express the vitamin D receptor (VDR) which mediates the biological effects of 1,25$(OH)_2$D at the cellular level by stimulating genomic or non-genomic responses [28]. For instance, studies have shown that 1,25$(OH)_2$D can inhibit renin expression through the interaction of the VDR with vitamin D response elements located in the promoter region of the renin gene [30]. Similarly, 1,25$(OH)_2$D can regulate the expression of over 200 genes, several of which are involved in cell growth and immunity [30]. Taken together, these mechanistic findings point to an important role for vitamin D as an autocrine/paracrine regulator of cell function. The investigation into these "non-classical" paracrine actions of vitamin D and their relation to human health is currently an active area of research. Moreover, the long-term programming effects of vitamin D may prove to be a consequence of its effects on extra-renal target tissues.

Potential Programming Effects of Vitamin D

At the beginning of the 20th century, it was well characterized that mothers with pelvic abnormalities gave birth to children who developed rickets; and that poor nutrition, lack of sunlight and the number of births contributed to the severity of the disease in both the mother and child [31]. Moreover, pregnant mothers who were administered cod liver oil, rich in vitamin A and vitamin D, had lower incidence or severity of rickets [31, 32]. Alfred Hess and Lester Unger, who examined a population of black women in New York where 90% of babies had rickets, revealed that higher doses (1620 mL) of cod liver oil prevented rickets better than lower doses (690 mL) [33, 34]. In this study, the duration of cod liver oil exposure also had a significant effect on rickets, with 6 months conferring greater protection against rickets than 4 months. Subsequently, a series of experiments by McMullen identified vitamin D as the anti-rachitic component of cod liver oil and provided preliminary evidence that vitamin D could modulate calcium and bone metabolism [35]. Subsequent studies showed that vitamin D status during development is positively associated with bone acquisition and peak bone mass, a major determinant of osteoporotic fractures [36-39]. In a longitudinal study, offspring whose mothers were vitamin D deficient (<27.5 nmol/L) during pregnancy had significantly lower whole body and lumbar spine bone mineral content at 9 years of age compared to those born to mothers who were vitamin D replete (>50 nmol/L); and children born to vitamin D insufficient (27.5-50 nmol/L) mothers during pregnancy had intermediate bone mineral accrual [38]. Similarly, Zamora et al [39] showed that Caucasian girls aged 7-9 years who received vitamin D supplementation during infancy had greater areal bone mineral density at the radius and proximal femur than the non-supplemented girls.

Evidence is now accumulating that vitamin D can affect the structural and functional development of many tissues aside from bone and thus may protect against several diseases [11]. According to the United Nations Standing Committee on Nutrition, a window of opportunity exists from pre-pregnancy to 24 months of childhood during which bioactive food components or vitamins can affect the development of an organism [40]. However, the mechanisms by which vitamin D affects programming of human health have not been extensively studied. It is possible that vitamin D may modulate human health in part through a process called metabolic imprinting [11]. This process is involved in fine tuning gene and protein expression during perinatal life, without directly altering the DNA sequence, to produce a phenotype that is best suited to survive in its predicted environment. However, if the environmental circumstances in later life are not as anticipated during perinatal development, the organism may be at risk of maladaptive physiology and ultimately disease [10].

The growth of the fetus is a dynamic process that is tightly controlled through multidirectional interactions between the mother, placenta and fetus. As such, the mother supplies nutrients and oxygen to the fetus through the placenta, which is formed in the fourth week of gestation. The placenta is perfused with maternal blood which allows 25(OH)D and oxygen to be transferred from the mother to the fetus [41]. It is thought that 25(OH)D crosses the hemochorial placenta readily [42] and that fetal 25(OH)D concentrations are approximately 87% of maternal concentrations [41, 43]. Thus, it is imperative that the mother is sufficient in vitamin D during pregnancy so that her developing offspring also possesses adequate vitamin D status during critical stages of development [42].

In contrast, the physiologically active metabolite 1,25$(OH)_2$D does not readily cross the placenta [44]. Instead, 1,25$(OH)_2$D is synthesized *in situ* by the placenta and fetal kidney which express the 1α-OHase enzyme that converts 25(OH)D to 1,25$(OH)_2$D [44]. It has been reported that there is an up-regulation in CYP27B1 expression during placental development, which increases the level of 1α-OHase and elevates the production of 1,25$(OH)_2$D [45, 46]. Moreover, Novakovic et al [47] demonstrated that the upstream promoter of placental CYP24A1 gene is hypermethylated, which represses 24-OHase transcription and thereby down-regulates 24,25$(OH)_2$D synthesis. This epigenetic decoupling of vitamin D feedback ensures that placental vitamin D activation exceeds clearance (i.e. 1,25$(OH)_2$D > 24,25$(OH)_2$D) during development and that vitamin D bioavailability is maximized at the fetomaternal interface [47]. As such, serum 1,25$(OH)_2$D concentrations are two-fold higher in pregnant women compared to non-pregnant or post-partum women [48, 49].

It is generally accepted that placental 1,25$(OH)_2$D enters both the maternal and fetal circulation but the mechanism of 1,25$(OH)_2$D uptake is poorly understood. Vitamin D and its metabolites [i.e. 25(OH)D, 1,25$(OH)_2$D and 24,25$(OH)_2$D] are hydrophobic and thus, are primarily transported in the blood bound to VDBPs, which act as a vitamin D reservoir and slow down the rate of metabolism [50, 51]. In both the mother and the fetus, total 1,25$(OH)_2$D concentrations increase by two-fold in the first trimester with more than 85% bound to VDBP [52]. However, the free hormone has only been shown to increase in the last trimester of pregnancy, the reason for which is not clearly understood [42].

It is widely assumed that the free hormone (i.e. non-protein bound) reflects the more biologically active form of vitamin D. Free 1,25$(OH)_2$D is carried through circulation by albumin and lipoprotein to the plasma membrane where it binds to VDR and stimulates genomic or non-genomic responses [51, 53]. In the genomic pathway, 1,25$(OH)_2$D binds with high affinity to the ligand binding domain of the VDR, which causes co-repressors to rapidly detach from the VDR. The ligand-bound VDR then forms a heterodimer with another receptor (i.e. retinoid X receptor) and the complex activates or represses gene transcription by binding to the vitamin D response element (VDRE) in the promoter regions of the gene [51]. Alternatively, in the non-genomic pathway, 1,25$(OH)_2$D binds to VDR associated with caveolae of the plasma membrane and then activates one or more signalling cascades (e.g.. protein kinase C, mitogen-activated protein kinases, phospholipase A_2 and phospholipase C) [51, 54, 55]. Each cascade has the potential to activate other signals, which can induce cellular changes by affecting the expression of the DNA in the nucleus or the activity of enzymes in the cytoplasm [51].

Vitamin D is a potent secosteroid hormone and its active form (1,25$(OH)_2$D) has diverse roles in regulating cell division, apoptosis, immune function and secretion of placental hormones (i.e. human chorionic gonadotropin, human placental lactogen, estradiol and progesterone) [51, 56]. As such, 1,25$(OH)_2$D aids in placental implantation, lowers the rate of maternal infection and supports fetal growth and development [51, 57, 58]. Each of these processes play a critical role in both short- and long-term programming of health. For example, 1,25$(OH)_2$D inhibits the release of Th1 cytokines including interferon-gamma, interleukin (IL) -2 and tumour necrosis factor-alpha (TNF-α) that alter the adaptive immune response and cause inflammation. Furthermore, 1,25$(OH)_2$D increases the release of Th2 cytokines (i.e. IL-4-6, IL-9, IL-10 and IL-13) that generate protective immunity [51, 57, 58]. Such immunomodulation may prevent rejection of the implanted embryo and reduce the risk of preeclampsia and premature labour. Indeed, epidemiological data indicates that the rates of preeclampsia and premature labour are elevated during winter months when solar production of vitamin D is reduced [59], and among vitamin D deficient women [60, 61]. A Norwegian study showed that pregnant women who were supplemented with 400-600 IU of vitamin D/d had a 27% reduction in the risk of preeclampsia compared to non-supplemented controls [62]. In comparison to healthy controls, preeclamptic or premature children often have a smaller size at birth, which is also a risk factor for cardio-metabolic diseases and cancers. Thus, vitamin D is important in maintaining the quality of the intrauterine environment such that reduced vitamin D status during pregnancy produces prenatal constraints that predispose the infant to future non-communicable diseases.

Reports of maternal and neonatal vitamin D insufficiency during pregnancy are abundant with the most recent report indicating that 69% of pregnant women have suboptimal (<75 nmol/L) 25(OH) concentrations [63]. Schroth et al [64] reviewed the prevalence of vitamin D deficiency during pregnancy and found that 35 out of 76 published studies reported highly deficient (<25 nmoL/L) 25(OH)D levels. These findings are worrisome because vitamin D deficiency can result in maternal secondary hyperparathyroidism, which can lead to transitory hypocalcemia and hyperparathyroidism in the neonate. It can also disrupt the maternal immune system and alter maternal peripheral blood gene expression and post-transcriptional regulation [65]. Recently, a study using microarray analyses correlated maternal plasma 25[OH]D concentrations in early pregnancy with transcriptional and post-transcriptional gene regulation at the mRNA and microRNA level, respectively [65]. Findings revealed differential expression in 305 genes (299 up-regulated and 6 down-regulated) and 11 microRNAs (10 down-regulated and 1 up-regulated) between women with low (<64 nmol/L) compared to high (≥79 nmol/L) 25[OH]D concentrations. These differentially expressed genes influence a wide range of cellular functions, including organ and system development, inflammation, energy production, cell signalling and DNA replication, recombination and repair [65]. Abnormalities in one or more of these cellular processes can be associated with cancer, diabetes, inflammation/immune-related disturbances, and other metabolic disorders [65]. Future work focused on unravelling the relation between vitamin D induced gene transcription and post-transcriptional regulation may help uncover the biological mechanisms involved in vitamin D-mediated pathophysiologic processes. Moreover, such research may shed light on how early feeding practices can be modified to minimize the risk of disease at adulthood.

Vitamin D, Imprinting and Cancer?

Due to its wide ranging effects in gene expression, it has been hypothesized that vitamin D deficiency in early life can increase risk of cancer at adulthood. Cancer is one of the most common diseases in North America and accounts for nearly 1 in every 4 deaths [66]. In 2010, it was estimated that over 1.5 billion new cases of cancer will be diagnosed and half a million cancer deaths will be reported in the US alone [66]. All cancers involve the malfunction of genes that control cell growth and division, but only 5% of cancers are caused by inherited genes [66]. In most cases, genetic damage is caused by internal factors (i.e. hormones, immune conditions or nutrient metabolism) or external factors (i.e. tobacco, chemicals, toxins, infectious organisms or radiation), which may act together or sequentially to initiate or promote carcinogenesis. Research from ecological, cross-sectional, and observational data indicates that solar UV-B exposure, as an index of cutaneous vitamin D photo-production, is inversely correlated with incidence and mortality rates of various cancers, including bladder, breast, colon, endometrial esophageal, gallbladder, gastric, lung, ovarian, pancreatic, prostate, rectal, renal, melanoma, Hodgkin's and non-Hodgkin's lymphoma. These studies are powerful in that they can analyze the effect of cancer risk-modifying factors over the entire lifespan of an individual beginning *in utero* [67]. There is also evidence that higher vitamin D status at the time of cancer diagnosis is associated with increased survival rate [68, 69].

The mechanism for the potential antineoplastic effect of vitamin D includes pathways involved in cellular differentiation and proliferation, angiogenesis and metastasis [70]. Most cells express the VDR and can transactivate or repress gene transcription upon $1,25(OH)_2D$ exposure by modulating G_0/G_1 arrest [71]. The exact sequence of events between VDR hetero-dimerization and transcriptional modulation has not been fully characterized but, it is clear that alterations in the relative expression and/or cellular distribution of vitamin D regulated genes can affect many molecular processes that mediate cancer initiation, development and progression. Moreover, studies have shown that 1,25$(OH)_2$D inhibits proliferation in various cell types by inducing cell cycle inhibitors that prevent the transition from the G1 to the S phase of the cell cycle. Also, 1,25$(OH)_2$D can promote differentiation by changing the expression of growth factors and cytokines [51]. VDR knockout mice exposed to carcinogens exhibit increased cellular proliferation and develop cancer earlier than the respective controls [70]. There is also evidence that 1,25$(OH)_2$D inhibits cell growth [72] and induces apoptosis [73, 74] by interfering with signalling pathways including tumor necrosis factor-β (TNF-β), epidemeral growth factor, insulin-like growth factor-I (IGF-I) and prostaglandins. Lastly, *in vitro* and *in vivo* models have demonstrated that 1,25$(OH)_2$D inhibits angiogenesis [75, 76] and tumour metastasis [70]. Despite progress in vitamin D and cancer research, there is a need to delineate the role of vitamin D in the prevention, progression and treatment of tissue-specific cancers.

Vitamin D, Imprinting and Prostate Cancer: Potential Mechanisms

Prostate cancer (PCa) is a major public health concern worldwide. It is the most common (nonskin) cancer among men in the Western world, affecting 1 in 6 American men. In 2010, there were an estimated 217,730 new cases of PCa and 32,050 deaths from PCa in the United States [77]. A strategy to prevent or reduce the risk of developing PCa is urgently needed. There is evidence that vitamin D may protect against PCa by regulating the expression of genes involved in prostate development and function, specifically, calbindin-D_{28K} ($CaBP_{28K}$) and testosterone.

During gestation, the fertilized egg undergoes a series of reproductive cell divisions to give rise to three germ layers (i.e. endoderm, mesoderm, and ectoderm) that mediate differentiation of various types of cells and are forerunners of all tissues and organs [11]. During this time, localized concentrations of vitamin D obtained from the maternal diet and body supply can interact with signalling molecules and modulate organ development. Animal studies indicate that defects in development or growth are not observed before weaning when vitamin D metabolism is reduced. However, significant alterations are observed in skeletal and reproductive tissues in these animals upon sexual maturation (post-weaning) [78-80], suggesting that vitamin D has long-term programming effects on organ development and function. For example, VDR knockout mice develop normally until weaning, however, post-weaning they fail to thrive, develop alopecia, hypocalcaemia, uterine hypoplasia and have impaired bone formation and folliculogenesis in reproductive organs [80]. Similarly, 1α-OHase deficient mice develop normally during early life but present with hypocalcaemia, secondary hyperparathyroidism, retarded growth, skeletal abnormalities and reduced fertility post-weaning [78, 79]. Moreover, studies indicate that vitamin D deficient animals are capable of reproducing but have markedly reduced success in mating [81, 82]. Vitamin D deficient male rats have a 45% lower mating ability (i.e. presence of sperm in the vaginal tract of the female) and a 73% lower fertility (successful conception) compared to vitamin D replete animals [82]. Litters from vitamin D deficient female rats were also shown to have reduced fertility indicating that vitamin D influences long-term programming of reproductive health [81, 83]. It remains unclear whether these reproductive effects are mediated by vitamin D directly or involve calcium regulation.

It is well documented that at the end of the foetal period, the male and female urogential systems are identical [84]. In the male embryo the paramesonephric ducts then degenerate and the uterovaginal canal grows into the urogenital sinus, contacts the posterior wall and migrates distally to the proximal part of the urethra. The increase in cellularity surrounding the urethra is the first sign of prostate formation. In the tenth week of gestation, androgens produced by the Leydig cells of the testes stimulate epithelial bud formation in the presumptive prostatic urethra leading to second phase budding and branching under mesodermal control [85, 86]. The Leydig cells also express $CaBP_{28K}$, which is a molecular marker for vitamin D action [83, 87]. Chickens fed a vitamin D deficient diet from postnatal day 1 to 8 weeks of age were shown to have significantly lower $CaBP_{28K}$ expression compared to vitamin D replete animals despite having normal calcium levels [83]. Cell culture studies indicate that low $CaBP_{28K}$ expression can increase apoptosis when exposed to environmental agents (i.e. dexamethasone and forskolin) that stimulate intracellular cAMP production [88].

Based on the literature to date, we hypothesize that vitamin D may reduce the risk of PCa by stimulating $CaBP_{28K}$, which buffers calcium fluxes and suppresses cell death. There is also evidence that vitamin D may regulate testosterone [89], a male hormone that stimulates prostate gland development and maturation. In the 11th week of gestation, mesenchymal cells differentiate into smooth muscle, fibroblasts and blood vessels, while the epithelial cords and cellular end buds form acini [84]. By the 14th week of gestation, peak testosterone concentrations are reached in the embryo and this rise in testosterone stimulates epithelial cells to differentiate in the proximal region of the larger ducts and progress distally. By the end of the 15th week, the secretory cells are functional, the basal cell populations have formed and neuroendocrine cells have developed. The prostate gland matures while embryonic testosterone levels are high but enters a quiescent state as testosterone levels fall during the third trimester. This quiescent state persists until puberty, at which point testosterone levels increase and the epithelium proliferates, giving rise to the complex folding seen in the mature gland. During puberty the prostate gland doubles in size, androgen receptors (AR) are expressed in the epithelial cells and the full secretory phenotype is established. In the fifth decade of life, when testosterone begin to decline the prostate gland undergoes a period of involution, which can lead to hypertrophy or cancer. Rats exposed to a calcium and vitamin D deprived diet with low phosphorus (0.4%) from day 1 of pregnancy to 60 days postpartum have significantly reduced testosterone (8.11 ± 5.64 ng/dl vs. 168.00 ± 41.14 ng/dl) levels compared to animals fed the normal diet [90]. Further research is needed to determine whether these reductions in testosterone concentrations can alter prostate gland development, maturation or function.

Epidemiological Evidence

No studies have examined the effects of vitamin D exposure in early life on risk of developing PCa. Known major risk factors for PCa include age, race, and geography. The risk of developing PCa increases with age, as 80-90% of all PCa diagnoses and mortalities occur in men over 65 years of age. PCa is considerably more common in Black men compared to other races. Moreover, Black men are more likely to be diagnosed at an advanced stage, and are more than twice as likely to die of PCa than White men [77]. Finally, several studies have demonstrated geographic patterns in PCa incidence and mortality such that these rates are higher in northern latitudes.

In 1990, Schwartz hypothesized that these major risk factors for PCa (i.e. age, race, geography) are all associated with decreased synthesis of vitamin D [91]. The elderly are frequently vitamin D deficient for several reasons including reduced exposure to sunlight [92] and the decreased capacity of older skin to generate vitamin D [94]. In terms of race, the higher melanin content in darker skin blocks the UV-B light required for vitamin D synthesis [94], which often results in lower serum 25(OH)D levels among pigmented races [95]. Inadequate sunlight/UV-B exposure has been consistently implicated as a risk factor for PCa incidence and mortality in several studies. Table 2 summarizes the epidemiological studies on the association between sunlight exposure and PCa risk. Hanchette et al [96] demonstrated that age-adjusted PCa mortality rates in the US are inversely proportional to UV radiation, the principle source of vitamin D. These findings were supported by data from the NHANES I cohort, which demonstrated that lower risk of PCa was significantly associated with residence in the South US at baseline (RR = 0.68, CI = 0.41-1.13), state of longest residence in the South US (RR = 0.62, CI = 0.40-0.95), and high solar radiation in the state of birth (RR = 0.49, CI = 0.30-0.79) [97].

A similar epidemiological study reported that, in addition to sun exposure in adulthood, early-life sun exposure was associated with a significant 51% reduced risk of PCa [98]. Of note, this study suggests that vitamin D exposure during early life could influence subsequent PCa risk later in life. Lastly, PCa patients were found to have better prognosis (15-50%) if they were diagnosed with PCa during the summer or autumn compared to the winter months [68]. Similar geographic patterns in cancer risk and mortality have been demonstrated for other cancers, including those of the colon and breast [99-102].

The association between dietary intake of vitamin D and PCa is less consistent as shown in Table 2. A prospective study of 3612 men followed for 8-10 years found no association between vitamin D intake and PCa risk [103]. A meta-analysis of 45 observational studies indicated that dietary vitamin D intake (<400 IU/d) was not related to PCa risk [104]. However, Ahn et al [105] reported a 40% reduction in PCa risk with >600 IU of supplemental vitamin D compared to no supplements. These findings suggest that vitamin D may be protective against PCa only when dietary consumption levels exceed recommended intakes.

Several studies have evaluated PCa risk in relation to serum levels of vitamin D metabolites, but the results have been mixed (Table 2). Corder et al [106] showed that PCa risk decreased with higher levels of $1,25(OH)_2D$, especially in those men with low 25(OH)D (OR = 0.15, CI = 0.03-0.85). A nested case-control study from Finland found that PCa risk was more than 3 times higher among young men (<52 years) with the lowest serum 25(OH)D (≤40 nmol/L) concentrations compared to older men (>51 years) [108].

Table 2. Summary of selected epidemiological studies linking sunlight exposure, vitamin D intake, and serum vitamin D metabolites to prostate cancer risk

First author, year, place	Study design	No. of cases/controls (cohort)	RR (95% CI), P-value	Conclusions
Sunlight exposure and PCa risk				
Hanchette, 1992, US [96]	Ecological	N/A Epidemiological index: n = 220 UV count: n = 3069 Latitude: n = 3073	Epidemiological index: r = -0.25, P < 0.0002 UV count: r = -0.15, P < 0.0001 Latitude: r = 0.19, P < 0.0001	PCa morality exhibits a north-south trend, with lower rates in the South. UV-B radiation may inhibit the development of clinical PCa.
John, 2004, US [97]	Cohort	153/3414	High solar radiation at longest residence: 0.62 (0.40-0.95) High solar radiation at place of birth: 0.49 (0.30-0.79)	Sunlight exposure reduces risk of PCa and has important implications for PCa prevention.
John, 2007, US [98]	Cohort	161/3367	High solar radiation in state of birth: 0.49 (0.27-0.90) Frequent recreational sun exposure in adulthood: 0.47 (0.23-0.99)	Sun exposure in both early life and adulthood protects against PCa.
Robsahm, 2004, Norway [68]	Cohort	16,457 PCa deaths 39,583 PCa cases	Summer diagnosis: 0.80 (0.75-0.84) Fall diagnosis: 0.70 (0.66-0.74)	Higher UV radiation at the time of diagnosis (i.e. summer, fall) may improve prognosis of PCa.
Vitamin D intake and PCa risk				
Tseng, 2005, US [103]	Prospective cohort	131/3612	0.6 (0.3-1.2), P = 0.16	After adjustment for calcium intake, vitamin D was not associated with PCa risk.
Huncharek, 2008, US [104]	Review meta-analysis	26769	1.16 (0.98-1.38)	Dietary intake of vitamin D was not related to PCa risk.
Ahn, 2007, US [105]	Cohort	1910/29509	0.61 (0.41-0.89), P = 0.05	PCa risk tended to decrease with greater vitamin D from supplemental sources, with a 40% reduction in men who used >600 IU of vitamin D daily compared to men not using vitamin D supplements.

First author, year, place	Study design	No. of cases/controls (cohort)	RR (95% CI), P-value	Conclusions
Serum vitamin D metabolites and PCa risk				
Corder, 1993, US [106]	Case-control	181/181	0.15 (0.03-0.85)	PCa risk decreased with higher levels of 1,25$(OH)_2D$ especially in men with low levels of 25(OH)D.
Ahonen, 2000, Finland [107]	Nested case-control	149/566	1.7 (1.0-3.0), P = 0.01	Low levels of 25(OH)D were associated with an increased risk for subsequent earlier exposure and more aggressive development of PCa, especially before andropause.
Tretli, 2009, Norway [69]	Cohort	19/52	25(OH)D (50-80 mol/L): 0.33 (0.14-0.77) 25(OH)D (>80 nmol/L): 0.16 (0.05-0.43)	Serum 25(OH)D may be involved in disease progression and is a potential marker of prognosis in patients with PCa.
Ahn, 2008, US [109]	Nested case-control	749/781	1.08 (0.77-1.53), P = 0.15	Serum 25(OH)D was not associated with risk for non-aggressive PCa.
Gann, 1996, US [110]	Nested case-control	232/414	25(OH)D: 0.92 (0.56-1.50), P = 0.82 1,25$(OH)_2D$: 0.88 (0.53-1.45), P = 0.50	Higher circulating levels of total or free vitamin D metabolites did not reduce PCa risk.
Platz, 2004, US [111]	Case-control	460/460	25(OH)D: 1.19 (0.79-1.79), P = 0.59 1,25$(OH)_2D$: 1.25 (0.82-1.90), P = 0.16	There was no inverse association between plasma 25(OH)D or 1,25$(OH)_2D$ concentrations and the incidence of PCa.
Tuohimaa, 2004, Norway, Finland, Sweden [112]	Longitudinal nested case-control	622/1451	Lowest 25(OH)D: 1.5 (0.8-2.7) Highest 25(OH)D: 1.7 (1.1-2.4)	Both low (<19 nmol/L) and high (>80 nmol/L) serum 25(OH)D are associated with higher PCa risk.

Recently, Tretli et al [69] reported that PCa patients with medium (50-80 nmol/L) and high (>80 nmol/L) 25(OH)D concentrations had a 67% and 84% lower risk of death from PCa, respectively, compared to those with low (<50 nmol/L) 25(OH)D concentrations. Vieth et al [109] showed that among PCa patients (untreated, low-grade), the rise in prostate specific antigen (PSA), the most widely-used clinical biomarker of PCa, was slower in the spring and summer when serum 25(OH)D levels were rising. However, other studies failed to demonstrate a correlation between PCa risk and vitamin D status [109-111]. Tuohimaa et al [112] reported a U-shaped risk curve, whereby both low (<19 nmol/L) and high (>80 nmol/L) serum 25(OH)D concentrations were associated with higher PCa risk. Vieth [113, 114] hypothesized that this phenomenon may be explained by the potentially detrimental consequences of dynamically fluctuating 25(OH)D supplies that occur with seasons at high latitudes.

Experimental Evidence

Considerable evidence implicates the prostate as a target organ for vitamin D. Skowronski et al [115] reported VDR expression in LNCaP, PC-3, and DU 145 PCa cell lines, as well as growth inhibition by $1,25(OH)_2D$ (1-100 nmol/L) treatment amounting to ~60%, ~40-50%, and ~10% of controls, respectively. Similarly $1,25(OH)_2D$-induced growth arrest (ED_{50} = 0.25-1 nmol/L) was demonstrated in primary epithelial cells derived from normal, benign prostate hyperplasia and cancerous regions of prostate obtained during prostatectomy [116].

Numerous studies have reported 1α-OHase expression in the prostate, supporting the chemotherapeutic utility of 25(OH)D through local prostatic conversion to $1,25(OH)_2D$ [117-120]. Growth of primary cultures of normal [118] and malignant [117] prostate cells was inhibited by physiological concentrations of 25(OH)D (i.e. 100 nmol/L) at an equal potency to pharmacological (and less safe) doses of $1,25(OH)_2D$. However, this therapeutic approach may be limited because some PCa cell lines exhibit lower 1α-OHase [119] and higher 24-OHase [121] expression, which reduces the availability of prostatic $1,25(OH)_2D$. Recently, Tokar and Webber [122, 123] reported that normal and malignant prostate epithelial cell lines constitutively express 25-OHase (CYP27A1), an enzyme capable of directly converting vitamin D into 25(OH)D and $1,25(OH)_2D$. Treatment of these cells with physiological levels of vitamin D_3 inhibited growth, induced differentiation, and decreased invasion by upregulating VDR, retinoid X receptor, and AR [122, 123]. The unique ability of prostate to locally produce $1,25(OH)_2D$ from circulating vitamin D as well as paracrine $1,25(OH)_2D$ synthesis by neighbouring normal PCa cells could circumvent the lower 1α-OHase and higher 24-OHase expression observed in prostate carcinoma. Taken together, these findings suggest that high-dose vitamin D can be an effective agent for PCa treatment and prevention.

The *in vivo* effects of vitamin D in PCa animal models have been mostly studied using $1,25(OH)_2D$ or synthetic vitamin D analogs. Blutt et al [124] showed that intraperitoneal injections of the vitamin D analog EB1089 substantially reduced the growth of LNCaP tumour xenografts in nude mice, without inducing hypercalcemia. Studies of the highly metastatic MAT LyLu Dunning tumour model in rats showed that $1,25(OH)_2D$, as well as the Ro23-6760 and EB1089 vitamin D analogs, inhibited tumour growth and reduced lung metastases in these animals [125, 126]. Xue et al [127] demonstrated that a high fat, low calcium, and low vitamin D diet fed to rats resulted in hyperproliferation of the prostate epithelium, a process which was subsequently inhibited by increasing levels of calcium and vitamin D in the rat diet.

There appear to be multiple genomic and non-genomic mechanisms by which $1,25(OH)_2D$ induces growth inhibition, including the previously mentioned effects on cell cycle arrest, apoptosis, metastasis, and angiogenesis. In one study, treatment of LNCaP cells with $1,25(OH)_2D$ increased the expression of CDK inhibitor p21 and decreased CDK2 activity, leading to a reduction in phosphorylation of the retinoblastoma protein and repression of E2F transcriptional activity, resulting in G1 arrest of the cells [128]. The elevations in p21 may be mediated indirectly by $1,25(OH)_2D$ induced upregulation of insulin-like growth factor binding protein-3 expression [129]. Blutt et al [130] demonstrated evidence of apoptosis in LNCaP cells exposed to $1,25(OH)_2D$, including the downregulation of the pro-apoptotic proteins Bcl-2 and Bcl-X_L. In prostate epithelial cell lines, $1,25(OH)_2D$ or its precursors increased expression of PSA [69, 131], a differentiation marker, and decreased expression of vimentin, a de-differentiation indicator [122], in part due to upregulation of AR. Furthermore, $1,25(OH)_2D$, along with its analogs and precursors, have also been shown to reduce markers of tumour invasion and metastasis, including matrix metalloproteinases [122, 132] and cell-surface integrins [133]. Studies have indicated that $1,25(OH)_2D$ can inhibit tumour cell-induced angiogenesis in mice [134] and reduce the angiogenic signaling molecule angiopoietin-2 in tumour-derived endothelial cells [135]. Lastly, cDNA microarray analyses have revealed several novel putative vitamin D target genes in prostate cells including MAP kinase phosphatase 5 and superoxide dismutase 2, which are involved in protection from oxidative stress, metallothionein cell survival factors, tumour necrosis factor, and several others [136, 137].

Clinical Trial Evidence

A small number of human intervention studies have examined the safety and efficacy of vitamin D treatment in PCa. However, most of these investigations used $1,25(OH)_2D$ or its analogs, rather than dietary vitamin D or vitamin D supplements, and have yielded mixed results. A small phase II dose-escalation trial of oral $1,25(OH)_2D$ (0.5-1.5 μg/d) in 14 patients with advanced metastatic androgen-independent PCa (AIPCa) reported no responses (>50% reduction in PSA or >30% reduction in tumour mass) with treatment [139]. Gross et al [139] conducted a pilot trial of increasing doses of $1,25(OH)_2D$ (0.5-2.5 μg/d) in 7 patients with early recurrent PCa following radiation or prostatectomy. This study found a substantial reduction in the rate of PSA rise in all patients, suggesting that $1,25(OH)_2D$ therapy could be effective in slowing PCa progression. However, in both of these early trials, hypercalciuria or hypercalcemia limited the clinical utility of $1,25(OH)_2D$ in PCa therapy.

More recent clinical trials have attempted to circumvent the calcemic side effects of $1,25(OH)_2D$ administration by altering its dosing regimen or employing less calcemic analogs. Beer et al [140] showed that high-dose weekly oral $1,25(OH)_2D$ (0.5 ug/kg) for a median of 10 months was safe (no hypercalcemia or renal calculi was detected) in PCa patients with rising PSA after therapy, although it did not achieve the endpoint of 50% reduction in PSA. DN-101 (Novacea Inc., San Francisco, CA), a proprietary formulation of high-dose $1,25(OH)_2D$ (45 μg weekly), was shown to be safe and able to attain the high systemic exposures (>1 nmol/L of 1,25$(OH)_2$D) required for anti-tumour activity [141, 142]. In the AIPCa Study of Calcitriol Enhancing Taxotere (ASCENT) phase II trial, the addition of DN-101 to weekly docetaxel was associated with a significant 33% reduction in the risk of death, although this combination did not produce a significant improvement in PSA response [143]. The improved survival led to a phase III trial of this regimen (ASCENT-2), in which survival was a primary endpoint. Unfortunately, ASCENT-2 was terminated abruptly after enrolment of 900 men due to excess number of deaths in the DN-101 arm. It is unclear whether the negative findings of ASCENT-2 were related to 1,25$(OH)_2$D *per se* or flawed study design [144]. Of note, ASCENT-2 had serious methodological issues, including: 1) the docetaxel dosing regimen in the DN-101 arm (weekly, 36 mg/sqm) was different and shown by other trials to be inferior to that of the control group (every 3 weeks, 75 mg/sqm); this study design violates one of the primary tenets of RCT design; and 2) the dose was selected based more on convenience than RCT substantiation [i.e. no maximum-tolerated dose (MTD) or optimal dose of DN-101 for PCa therapy has been defined to date].

Analogs of 1,25$(OH)_2$D exhibit an improved safety profile over 1,25$(OH)_2$D, however, their clinical efficacy in PCa has not been confirmed. A phase I/II trial of paricalcitol (Abbot Pharmaceuticals, Abbott Park, IL) in AIPCa patients did not show a response to treatment (i.e. PSA decline), although paricalcitol did reduce PTH, which was inversely associated with survival [145]. Similarly, phase II trials of doxercalciferol alone [146] or with docetaxel [147] failed to show objective responses in PSA or survival in AIPCa. Other vitamin D analogs, including seocalcitol (EB-1089; LEO Pharma, Ballerup, Denmark), inecalcitol (Hybrigenics, Paris, France), 22-oxa-calcitriol, calcipotriol (LEO Pharma), KH1060 (LEO Pharma), and R024-5531 are also being investigated as potential anticancer drugs.

The limited success of clinical trials of vitamin D-based compounds in PCa may relate to the choice of the therapeutic agent itself. To date, most studies have focused on the anticancer capacity of 1,25$(OH)_2$D or its analogs, but these require pharmacological doses and careful monitoring of calcium levels. However, preclinical evidence suggests that physiological levels of nutrient vitamin D_3 can exert similar antiproliferative effects as supraphysiological 1,25$(OH)_2$D concentrations without inducing calcemic side effects (see section on experimental evidence). In 2005, Woo et al [148] described the first clinical trial evaluating the efficacy of nutrient vitamin D_3 (2 000 IU/d) in 15 patients with recurrent PCa. Vitamin D_3 treatment decreased or stabilized PSA values in 9 patients for as long as 21 months of follow-up, delaying the implementation of androgen ablation. Furthermore, there was a statistically significant reduction in the rate of PSA rise after vitamin D_3 administration. Overall, 14 out of 15 patients had a prolonged PSA doubling time, which increased significantly from 14.3 to 25 months after commencing vitamin D_3 supplementation The positive findings from this pilot trial led to a phase II randomized trial (currently underway) of higher doses of oral vitamin D_3 [40 000, 10 000, or 400 (control) IU/d] administered preoperatively to early-stage PCa patients undergoing radical prostatectomy. The major outcomes of this ongoing study are immunohistochemical markers of prostate cell proliferation and vitamin D metabolite concentrations in prostate tissue (ClinicalTrials.gov Identifier: NCT00741364).

Conclusion

Evidence is accumulating that vitamin D is a critical modulator of human health, and that maternal vitamin D inadequacy may alter fetal development and predispose the individual to lifelong health problems that may include some metabolic diseases and possibly several types of cancer [11]. Many non-renal tissues locally produce the active vitamin D hormone and express vitamin D receptors and thus, can mediate genomic and non-genomic responses. As a result, vitamin D may have effects well beyond extracellular calcium and phosphate homeostasis. To date, studies have shown that vitamin D regulates the expression of more than 200 genes including calbindin-D_{28K} ($CaBP_{28K}$) and testosterone, which are involved in prostate maturation and function. Moreover, due to its wide ranging effects in gene expression, it has been hypothesized that vitamin D deficiency in early life as well as throughout life can increase the risk of prostate cancer at adulthood. To date, no studies have examined the effects of vitamin D exposure in early life on risk of developing PCa. A small number of human intervention studies have examined the safety and efficacy of vitamin D treatment in PCa. However, most of these investigations used $1,25(OH)_2D$ or its analogs and have yielded mixed results. Future research is needed to determine the role of vitamin D in prostate cancer and to form the basis for public health action.

Future Research Directions

Vitamin D remains an exciting area of research in disease epidemiology, prevention, and therapy. Definitive results from clinical studies are needed to support the persuasive epidemiological and experimental data reported to date. In particular, the optimal agent (i.e. nutrient vitamin D_3, its metabolites, or analogs), dose, and route of administration that provide maximal benefit specific to PCa prevention and therapy require further investigation. Given the substantial molecular heterogeneity in PCa, design of future studies should also consider the genetic variability in metabolic and functional responses to vitamin D dosing. The combination of vitamin D with other agents, including chemotherapeutic drugs, catabolic (i.e. 24-hydroxylase) inhibitors, soy isoflavones (e.g. genistein), retinoids, glucocorticoids, and other VDR ligands [144, 149] is a compelling strategy being tested that could yield synergistic efficacy in cancer prevention and therapy. Moreover, identification of critical windows during which vitamin D can prevent and/or treat disease is imperative for minimizing the risk of later disease and for implementing public health programs.

References

[1] Dorner, G., Perinatal hormone levels and brain organization., in Anatomical neuroendocrinology, W.E. Stumpf and L.D. Grand, Editors. 1975, Karger: Basel. p. 245-52.

[2] Koletzko, B., Developmental origins of adult disease: Barker's or Dorner's hypothesis? *Am. J. Hum. Biol.*, 2005. 17(3): p. 381-2.

[3] Barker, D.J., et al., Growth in utero, blood pressure in childhood and adult life, and mortality from cardiovascular disease. *BMJ,* 1989. 298(6673): p. 564-7.
[4] Soder, O., Perinatal imprinting by estrogen and adult prostate disease. *Proc. Natl. Acad. Sci. USA,* 2005. 102(5): p. 1269-70.
[5] Barker, D.J., et al., The surface area of the placenta and hypertension in the offspring in later life. *Int. J. Dev. Biol.*, 2010. 54(2-3): p. 525-30.
[6] Godfrey, K.M. and D.J. Barker, Maternal nutrition in relation to fetal and placental growth. *Eur. J. Obstet. Gynecol. Reprod. Biol.*, 1995. 61(1): p. 15-22.
[7] Dicke, J.M., Poor obstetrical outcome in Clinical Obstetrics, C.J. Pauerstein, Editor. 1987, Churchill Livingstone: Edinburgh. p. 421-39.
[8] Barker, D.J., Fetal nutrition and cardiovascular disease in later life. *Br. Med. Bull*, 1997. 53(1): p. 96-108.
[9] Barker, D.J., et al., Abnormal liver growth in utero and death from coronary heart disease. *BMJ*, 1995. 310(6981): p. 703-4.
[10] Burdge, G.C. and K.A. Lillycrop, Nutrition, epigenetics, and developmental plasticity: implications for understanding human disease. *Annu. Rev. Nutr.*, 2010. 30: p. 315-39.
[11] Kaludjerovic, J. and R. Vieth, Relationship between vitamin D during perinatal development and health. *J. Midwifery Womens Health*, 2010. 55(6): p. 550-60.
[12] Vieth, R., Effects of vitamin D on bone and natural selection of skin color: How much vitamin D nutrition are we talking about?, in Bone loss and osteoporosis: An anthropological perspective S.C. Agarwal and S.D. Stout, Editors. 2003, Kluwer Academic/Pleunum Publishers: New York.
[13] Hollis, B.W. and C.L. Wagner, Assessment of dietary vitamin D requirements during pregnancy and lactation. *Am. J. Clin. Nutr.*, 2004. 79(5): p. 717-26.
[14] Tsiaras, W.G. and M.A. Weinstock, Factors influencing vitamin d status. *Acta Derm. Venereol.*, 2011. 91(2): p. 115-24.
[15] Ovesen, L., C. Brot, and J. Jakobsen, Food contents and biological activity of 25-hydroxyvitamin D: a vitamin D metabolite to be reckoned with? *Ann. Nutr. Metab.*, 2003. 47(3-4): p. 107-13.
[16] Institute of Medicine, Food and Nutrition Board. Dietary intake assessment in Dietary reference intakes: calcium and vitamin D. **C. A. Ross, C.L. Taylor,A.L. Yaktine, H.B. Del Valle, Editors.** 2011, National Academies Press: Washington, DC. p. 457-478.
[17] Institute of Medicine, Food and Nutrition Board. Dietary reference intakes for calcium, phosphorus, magnesium, vitamin D, and fluoride. 1997, National Academies Press: Washington, DC.
[18] Institute of Medicine, Food and Nutrition Board, Dietary Reference Intakes for Calcium and Vitamin D. 2010, National Academies Press: Washington, DC.
[19] Taylor, S.N., C.L. Wagner, and B.W. Hollis, Vitamin D supplementation during lactation to support infant and mother. *J. Am. Coll Nutr.*, 2008. 27(6): p. 690-701.
[20] Vitamin D supplementation: Recommendations for Canadian mothers and infants. *Paediatr Child Health*, 2007. 12(7): p. 583-98.
[21] Jones, G., S.A. Strugnell, and H.F. DeLuca, Current understanding of the molecular actions of vitamin D. *Physiol Rev*, 1998. 78(4): p. 1193-231.
[22] Ponchon, G., A.L. Kennan, and H.F. DeLuca, "Activation" of vitamin D by the liver. *J. Clin. Invest.*, 1969. 48(11): p. 2032-7.

[23] Kimball, S., H. Fuleihan Gel, and R. Vieth, Vitamin D: a growing perspective. *Crit. Rev. Clin. Lab. Sci.*, 2008. 45(4): p. 339-414.
[24] Bischoff-Ferrari, H.A., et al., Estimation of optimal serum concentrations of 25-hydroxyvitamin D for multiple health outcomes. *Am. J. Clin. Nutr.*, 2006. 84(1): p. 18-28.
[25] Holick, M.F., Sunlight and vitamin D for bone health and prevention of autoimmune diseases, cancers, and cardiovascular disease. *Am. J. Clin. Nutr.*, 2004. 80(6 Suppl): p. 1678S-88S.
[26] McGrath, J., Does 'imprinting' with low prenatal vitamin D contribute to the risk of various adult disorders? *Med. Hypotheses*, 2001. 56(3): p. 367-71.
[27] Zehnder, D., et al., Extrarenal expression of 25-hydroxyvitamin d(3)-1 alpha-hydroxylase. *J. Clin. Endocrinol. Metab.*, 2001. 86(2): p. 888-94.
[28] Holick, M.F., Vitamin D: A millenium perspective. *J Cell Biochem*, 2003. 88(2): p. 296-307.
[29] Li, Y.C., et al., 1,25-Dihydroxyvitamin D(3) is a negative endocrine regulator of the renin-angiotensin system. *J. Clin. Invest*, 2002. 110(2): p. 229-38.
[30] Holick, M.F., Vitamin D deficiency. *N. Engl. J. Med.*, 2007. 357(3): p. 266-81.
[31] Maxwell, J.P., Further studies in adult rickets (Osteomalacia) and foetal rickets: (Section of Obstetrics and Gynaecology). *Proc. R. Soc. Med.*, 1935. 28(3): p. 265-300.
[32] Chick, D.H., Study of rickets in Vienna 1919-1922. *Med. Hist*, 1976. 20(1): p. 41-51.
[33] Rajakumar, K. and S.B. Thomas, Reemerging nutritional rickets: a historical perspective. *Arch. Pediatr. Adolesc. Med.*, 2005. 159(4): p. 335-41.
[34] Hess, A.F. and L.J. Unger, Prophylactic therapy for rickets in a Negro community. *JAMA*, 1917. 69: p. 1583.
[35] McCollum, E.V., et al., Studies on experimental rickets, XXI: an experimental demonstration of the existence of a vitamin which promotes calcium deposition.. *J. Biol. Chem.*, 1922. 53: p. 293-312.
[36] Heaney, R.P., et al., Peak bone mass. *Osteoporos Int.*, 2000. 11(12): p. 985-1009.
[37] Eisman, J.A., et al., Peak bone mass and osteoporosis prevention. *Osteoporos Int.*, 1993. 3 Suppl 1: p. 56-60.
[38] Javaid, M.K., et al., Maternal vitamin D status during pregnancy and childhood bone mass at age 9 years: a longitudinal study. *Lancet,* 2006. 367(9504): p. 36-43.
[39] Zamora, S.A., et al., Vitamin D supplementation during infancy is associated with higher bone mineral mass in prepubertal girls. *J. Clin. Endocrinol. Metab.*, 1999. 84(12): p. 4541-4.
[40] United Nations Standing Committee on Nutrition, Double burden of malnutrition - A common agenda, in 33rd Annual Session of the Standing Committee on Nutrition 2006, United Nations: Geneva, Switzerland.
[41] Dent, C.E. and M.M. Gupta, Plasma 25-hydroxyvitamin-D-levels during pregnancy in Caucasians and in vegetarian and non-vegetarian Asians. *Lancet*, 1975. 2(7944): p. 1057-60.
[42] Kovacs, C.S., Vitamin D in pregnancy and lactation: maternal, fetal, and neonatal outcomes from human and animal studies. *Am. J. Clin. Nutr.*, 2008. 88(2): p. 520S-528S.
[43] Fleischman, A.R., et al., Maternal and fetal serum 1,25-dihydroxyvitamin D levels at term. *J. Pediatr*, 1980. 97(4): p. 640-2.

[44] Greer, F.R., 25-Hydroxyvitamin D: functional outcomes in infants and young children. *Am. J. Clin. Nutr.*, 2008. 88(2): p. 529S-533S.

[45] Barrera, D., et al., Calcitriol affects hCG gene transcription in cultured human syncytiotrophoblasts. *Reprod. Biol. Endocrinol.*, 2008. 6: p. 3.

[46] Evans, K.N., et al., Vitamin D and placental-decidual function. *J. Soc. Gynecol. Investig.*, 2004. 11(5): p. 263-71.

[47] Novakovic, B., et al., Placenta-specific methylation of the vitamin D 24-hydroxylase gene: implications for feedback autoregulation of active vitamin D levels at the fetomaternal interface. *J. Biol. Chem.*, 2009. 284(22): p. 14838-48.

[48] Kovacs, C.S. and H.M. Kronenberg, Maternal-fetal calcium and bone metabolism during pregnancy, puerperium, and lactation. *Endocr. Rev.*, 1997. 18(6): p. 832-872.

[49] Cross, N.A., et al., Calcium homeostasis and bone metabolism during pregnancy, lactation, and postweaning: a longitudinal study. *Am. J. Clin. Nutr.*, 1995. 61(3): p. 514-523.

[50] Cooke, N.E. and J.G. Haddad, Vitamin D binding protein (Gc-globulin). *Endocr. Rev.*, 1989. 10(3): p. 294-307.

[51] Shin, J.S., et al., Vitamin D effects on pregnancy and the placenta. Placenta, 2010. 31(12): p. 1027-34.

[52] Bikle, D.D., et al., Serum protein binding of 1,25-dihydroxyvitamin D: a reevaluation by direct measurement of free metabolite levels. *J. Clin. Endocrinol. Metab.*, 1985. 61(5): p. 969-75.

[53] Brown, A.J., A. Dusso, and E. Slatopolsky, Vitamin D. *Am. J. Physiol.*, 1999. 277(2 Pt 2): p. F157-75.

[54] Mizwicki, M.T. and A.W. Norman, The vitamin D sterol-vitamin D receptor ensemble model offers unique insights into both genomic and rapid-response signaling. *Sci. Signal*, 2009. 2(75): p. re4.

[55] Huhtakangas, J.A., et al., The vitamin D receptor is present in caveolae-enriched plasma membranes and binds 1 alpha,25(OH)2-vitamin D3 in vivo and in vitro. *Mol. Endocrinol.*, 2004. 18(11): p. 2660-71.

[56] Barrera, D., et al., Estradiol and progesterone synthesis in human placenta is stimulated by calcitriol. *J. Steroid Biochem. Mol. Biol.,* 2007. 103(3-5): p. 529-32.

[57] Zehnder, D., et al., The ontogeny of 25-hydroxyvitamin D(3) 1alpha-hydroxylase expression in human placenta and decidua. *Am. J. Pathol.*, 2002. 161(1): p. 105-14.

[58] Piccinni, M.P., et al., Role of hormone-controlled Th1- and Th2-type cytokines in successful pregnancy. *J. Neuroimmunol.*, 2000. 109(1): p. 30-3.

[59] Magnu, P. and A. Eskild, Seasonal variation in the occurrence of pre-eclampsia. *BJOG*, 2001. 108(11): p. 1116-9.

[60] Bodnar, L.M., et al., Maternal vitamin D deficiency increases the risk of preeclampsia. *J. Clin. Endocrinol. Metab.*, 2007. 92(9): p. 3517-22.

[61] Shand, A.W., et al., Maternal vitamin D status in pregnancy and adverse pregnancy outcomes in a group at high risk for pre-eclampsia. *BJOG,* 2010. 117(13): p. 1593-8.

[62] Haugen, M., et al., Vitamin D supplementation and reduced risk of preeclampsia in nulliparous women. *Epidemiology,* 2009. 20(5): p. 720-6.

[63] Ginde, A.A., et al., Vitamin D insufficiency in pregnant and nonpregnant women of childbearing age in the United States. *Am. J. Obstet. Gynecol.*, 2010. 202(5): p. 436 e1-8.

[64] Schroth, R.J., C.L. Lavelle, and M.E. Moffatt, Review of vitamin D deficiency during pregnancy: who is affected? *Int. J. Circumpolar Health*, 2005. 64(2): p. 112-20.

[65] Enquobahrie, D.A., et al., Global maternal early pregnancy peripheral blood mRNA and miRNA expression profiles according to plasma 25-hydroxyvitamin D concentrations. *J. Matern Fetal Neonatal Med.*, 2011.

[66] American Cancer Society (2011) Cancer Facts and Figures 2010. 1-62.

[67] Grant, W.B., UVB-Vitamin D-Cancer Hypothesis. *J. Am. Diet Assoc.*, 2011. 111(3): p. 365-6.

[68] Robsahm, T.E., et al., Vitamin D3 from sunlight may improve the prognosis of breast-, colon- and prostate cancer (Norway). *Cancer Causes Control*, 2004. 15(2): p. 149-58.

[69] Tretli, S., et al., Association between serum 25(OH)D and death from prostate cancer. *Br. J. Cancer*, 2009. 100(3): p. 450-4.

[70] Bouillon, R., et al., Vitamin D and human health: lessons from vitamin D receptor null mice. *Endocr. Rev.*, 2008. 29(6): p. 726-76.

[71] Jensen, S.S., et al., Inhibitory effects of 1alpha,25-dihydroxyvitamin D(3) on the G(1)-S phase-controlling machinery. *Mol. Endocrinol.*, 2001. 15(8): p. 1370-80.

[72] Moreno, J., et al., Mechanisms of vitamin D-mediated growth inhibition in prostate cancer cells: inhibition of the prostaglandin pathway. *Anticancer Res.*, 2006. 26(4A): p. 2525-30.

[73] Xie, S.P., S.Y. James, and K.W. Colston, Vitamin D derivatives inhibit the mitogenic effects of IGF-I on MCF-7 human breast cancer cells. *J. Endocrinol.,* 1997. 154(3): p. 495-504.

[74] McGuire, T.F., D.L. Trump, and C.S. Johnson, Vitamin D(3)-induced apoptosis of murine squamous cell carcinoma cells. Selective induction of caspase-dependent MEK cleavage and up-regulation of MEKK-1. *J. Biol. Chem.*, 2001. 276(28): p. 26365-73.

[75] Nakagawa, K., et al., 1 alpha,25-Dihydroxyvitamin D(3) is a preventive factor in the metastasis of lung cancer. *Carcinogenesis,* 2005. 26(2): p. 429-40.

[76] Majewski, S., et al., Vitamin D3 is a potent inhibitor of tumor cell-induced angiogenesis. *J. Investig. Dermatol. Symp. Proc.*, 1996. 1(1): p. 97-101.

[77] American Cancer Society, Prostate Cancer Overview. 2011.

[78] Panda, D.K., et al., Targeted ablation of the 25-hydroxyvitamin D 1alpha -hydroxylase enzyme: evidence for skeletal, reproductive, and immune dysfunction. *Proc. Natl. Acad. Sci. USA*, 2001. 98(13): p. 7498-503.

[79] Dardenne, O., et al., Targeted inactivation of the 25-hydroxyvitamin D(3)-1(alpha)-hydroxylase gene (CYP27B1) creates an animal model of pseudovitamin D-deficiency rickets. *Endocrinology*, 2001. 142(7): p. 3135-41.

[80] Yoshizawa, T., et al., Mice lacking the vitamin D receptor exhibit impaired bone formation, uterine hypoplasia and growth retardation after weaning. *Nat Genet*, 1997. 16(4): p. 391-6.

[81] Kwiecinksi, G.G., G.I. Petrie, and H.F. DeLuca, 1,25-Dihydroxyvitamin D3 restores fertility of vitamin D-deficient female rats. *Am. J. Physiol.*, 1989. 256(4 Pt 1): p. E483-7.

[82] Kwiecinski, G.G., G.I. Petrie, and H.F. DeLuca, Vitamin D is necessary for reproductive functions of the male rat. *J. Nutr.*, 1989. 119(5): p. 741-4.

[83] Inpanbutr, N., et al., Effect of vitamin D on testicular CaBP28K expression and serum testosterone in chickens. *Biol. Reprod.*, 1996. 54(1): p. 242-8.

[84] The urogenital system, in The developing human: clinically oriented embryology, K.L. Moore and T.V.N. Persuad, Editors. 2008, Saunders: Philadelphia.

[85] Cotton, L.M., M.K. O'Bryan, and B.T. Hinton, Cellular signaling by fibroblast growth factors (FGFs) and their receptors (FGFRs) in male reproduction. *Endocr. Rev.*, 2008. 29(2): p. 193-216.

[86] Takeda, H., I. Lasnitzki, and T. Mizuno, Analysis of prostatic bud induction by brief androgen treatment in the fetal rat urogenital sinus. *J. Endocrinol.*, 1986. 110(3): p. 467-70.

[87] Inpanbutr, N. and A.N. Taylor, Expression of calbindin-D28k in developing and growing chick testes. *Histochemistry*, 1992. 97(4): p. 335-9.

[88] Dowd, D.R., et al., Stable expression of the calbindin-D28K complementary DNA interferes with the apoptotic pathway in lymphocytes. *Mol. Endocrinol.,* 1992. 6(11): p. 1843-8.

[89] Oliveira, A.G., et al., Vitamin D3 and androgen receptors in testis and epididymal region of roosters (Gallus domesticus) as affected by epididymal lithiasis. *Anim. Reprod. Sci.*, 2008. 109(1-4): p. 343-55.

[90] Mitra, S.K., et al., Bone mineralization by OST-6 (OsteoCare), a herbomineral preparation, in experimentally induced rickets in rats. *Phytomedicine,* 2000. 7(4): p. 265-72.

[91] Schwartz, G.G. and B.S. Hulka, Is vitamin D deficiency a risk factor for prostate cancer? (Hypothesis). *Anticancer Res.*, 1990. 10(5A): p. 1307-11.

[92] Lamberg-Allardt, C., Vitamin D intake, sunlight exposure and 25-hydroxyvitamin D levels in the elderly during one year. *Ann Nutr Metab*, 1984. 28(3): p. 144-50.

[93] MacLaughlin, J. and M.F. Holick, Aging decreases the capacity of human skin to produce vitamin D3. *J. Clin. Invest*, 1985. 76(4): p. 1536-8.

[94] Matsuoka, L.Y., et al., Racial pigmentation and the cutaneous synthesis of vitamin D. *Arch. Dermatol.*, 1991. 127(4): p. 536-8.

[95] Gozdzik, A., et al., Low wintertime vitamin D levels in a sample of healthy young adults of diverse ancestry living in the Toronto area: associations with vitamin D intake and skin pigmentation. *BMC Public Health*, 2008. 8: p. 336.

[96] Hanchette, C.L. and G.G. Schwartz, Geographic patterns of prostate cancer mortality. Evidence for a protective effect of ultraviolet radiation. *Cancer,* 1992. 70(12): p. 2861-9.

[97] John, E.M., et al., Residential sunlight exposure is associated with a decreased risk of prostate cancer. *J. Steroid Biochem. Mol. Biol.*, 2004. 89-90(1-5): p. 549-52.

[98] John, E.M., J. Koo, and G.G. Schwartz, Sun exposure and prostate cancer risk: evidence for a protective effect of early-life exposure. *Cancer Epidemiol. Biomarkers Prev.*, 2007. 16(6): p. 1283-6.

[99] Emerson, J.C. and N.S. Weiss, Colorectal cancer and solar radiation. *Cancer Causes Control*, 1992. 3(1): p. 95-9.

[100] Garland, C.F. and F.C. Garland, Do sunlight and vitamin D reduce the likelihood of colon cancer? *Int. J. Epidemiol.*, 1980. 9(3): p. 227-31.

[101] Garland, F.C., et al., Geographic variation in breast cancer mortality in the United States: a hypothesis involving exposure to solar radiation. *Prev. Med.*, 1990. 19(6): p. 614-22.

[102] Gorham, E.D., F.C. Garland, and C.F. Garland, Sunlight and breast cancer incidence in the USSR. *Int. J. Epidemiol.*, 1990. 19(4): p. 820-4.
[103] Tseng, M., et al., Dairy, calcium, and vitamin D intakes and prostate cancer risk in the National Health and Nutrition Examination Epidemiologic Follow-up Study cohort. *Am. J. Clin. Nutr.*, 2005. 81(5): p. 1147-54.
[104] Huncharek, M., J. Muscat, and B. Kupelnick, Dairy products, dietary calcium and vitamin D intake as risk factors for prostate cancer: a meta-analysis of 26,769 cases from 45 observational studies. *Nutr. Cancer*, 2008. 60(4): p. 421-41.
[105] Ahn, J., et al., Dairy products, calcium intake, and risk of prostate cancer in the prostate, lung, colorectal, and ovarian cancer screening trial. *Cancer Epidemiol Biomarkers Prev.*, 2007. 16(12): p. 2623-30.
[106] Corder, E.H., et al., Vitamin D and prostate cancer: a prediagnostic study with stored sera. *Cancer Epidemiol. Biomarkers Prev.*, 1993. 2(5): p. 467-72.
[107] Ahonen, M.H., et al., Prostate cancer risk and prediagnostic serum 25-hydroxyvitamin D levels (Finland). *Cancer Causes Control*, 2000. 11(9): p. 847-52.
[108] Vieth, R., et al., Rise in prostate-specific antigen in men with untreated low-grade prostate cancer is slower during spring-summer. *Am. J. Ther.*, 2006. 13(5): p. 394-9.
[109] Ahn, J., et al., Serum vitamin D concentration and prostate cancer risk: a nested case-control study. *J. Natl. Cancer Inst.*, 2008. 100(11): p. 796-804.
[110] Gann, P.H., et al., Circulating vitamin D metabolites in relation to subsequent development of prostate cancer. Canc*er Epidemiol. Biomarkers Prev*, 1996. 5(2): p. 121-6.
[111] Platz, E.A., et al., Plasma 1,25-dihydroxy- and 25-hydroxyvitamin D and subsequent risk of prostate cancer. *Cancer Causes Control*, 2004. 15(3): p. 255-65.
[112] Tuohimaa, P., et al., Both high and low levels of blood vitamin D are associated with a higher prostate cancer risk: a longitudinal, nested case-control study in the Nordic countries. *Int. J. Cancer*, 2004. 108(1): p. 104-8.
[113] Vieth, R., Enzyme kinetics hypothesis to explain the U-shaped risk curve for prostate cancer vs. 25-hydroxyvitamin D in nordic countries. *Int. J. Cancer*, 2004. 111(3): p. 468; author reply 469.
[114] Vieth, R., How to optimize vitamin D supplementation to prevent cancer, based on cellular adaptation and hydroxylase enzymology. *Anticancer Res.,* 2009. 29(9): p. 3675-84.
[115] Skowronski, R.J., D.M. Peehl, and D. Feldman, Vitamin D and prostate cancer: 1,25 dihydroxyvitamin D3 receptors and actions in human prostate cancer cell lines. *Endocrinology*, 1993. 132(5): p. 1952-60.
[116] Peehl, D.M., et al., Antiproliferative effects of 1,25-dihydroxyvitamin D3 on primary cultures of human prostatic cells. *Cancer Res.*, 1994. 54(3): p. 805-10.
[117] Chen, T.C., et al., The in vitro evaluation of 25-hydroxyvitamin D3 and 19-nor-1alpha,25-dihydroxyvitamin D2 as therapeutic agents for prostate cancer. *Clin. Cancer Res.*, 2000. 6(3): p. 901-8.
[118] Barreto, A.M., et al., 25-Hydroxyvitamin D3, the prohormone of 1,25-dihydroxyvitamin D3, inhibits the proliferation of primary prostatic epithelial cells. *Cancer Epidemiol. Biomarkers Prev.*, 2000. 9(3): p. 265-70.

[119] Hsu, J.Y., et al., Reduced 1alpha-hydroxylase activity in human prostate cancer cells correlates with decreased susceptibility to 25-hydroxyvitamin D3-induced growth inhibition. *Cancer Res*, 2001. 61(7): p. 2852-6.
[120] Schwartz, G.G., et al., Human prostate cells synthesize 1,25-dihydroxyvitamin D3 from 25-hydroxyvitamin D3. *Cancer Epidemiol. Biomarkers Prev.*, 1998. 7(5): p. 391-5.
[121] Miller, G.J., et al., Vitamin D receptor expression, 24-hydroxylase activity, and inhibition of growth by 1alpha,25-dihydroxyvitamin D3 in seven human prostatic carcinoma cell lines. *Clin. Cancer Res.,* 1995. 1(9): p. 997-1003.
[122] Tokar, E.J. and M.M. Webber, Cholecalciferol (vitamin D3) inhibits growth and invasion by up-regulating nuclear receptors and 25-hydroxylase (CYP27A1) in human prostate cancer cells. *Clin. Exp. Metastasis*, 2005. 22(3): p. 275-84.
[123] Tokar, E.J. and M.M. Webber, Chemoprevention of prostate cancer by cholecalciferol (vitamin D3): 25-hydroxylase (CYP27A1) in human prostate epithelial cells. *Clin. Exp. Metastasis*, 2005. 22(3): p. 265-73.
[124] Blutt, S.E., et al., A calcitriol analogue, EB1089, inhibits the growth of LNCaP tumors in nude mice. *Cancer Res.*, 2000. 60(4): p. 779-82.
[125] Getzenberg, R.H., et al., Vitamin D inhibition of prostate adenocarcinoma growth and metastasis in the Dunning rat prostate model system. *Urology,* 1997. 50(6): p. 999-1006.
[126] Lokeshwar, B.L., et al., Inhibition of prostate cancer metastasis in vivo: a comparison of 1,23-dihydroxyvitamin D (calcitriol) and EB1089. *Cancer Epidemiol Biomarkers Prev*, 1999. 8(3): p. 241-8.
[127] Xue, L., et al., Influence of dietary calcium and vitamin D on diet-induced epithelial cell hyperproliferation in mice. *J. Natl. Cancer Inst.*, 1999. 91(2): p. 176-81.
[128] Zhuang, S.H. and K.L. Burnstein, Antiproliferative effect of 1alpha,25-dihydroxyvitamin D3 in human prostate cancer cell line LNCaP involves reduction of cyclin-dependent kinase 2 activity and persistent G1 accumulation. *Endocrinology,* 1998. 139(3): p. 1197-207.
[129] Boyle, B.J., et al., Insulin-like growth factor binding protein-3 mediates 1 alpha,25-dihydroxyvitamin d(3) growth inhibition in the LNCaP prostate cancer cell line through p21/WAF1. *J. Urol.*, 2001. 165(4): p. 1319-24.
[130] Blutt, S.E., et al., Calcitriol-induced apoptosis in LNCaP cells is blocked by overexpression of Bcl-2. *Endocrinology*, 2000. 141(1): p. 10-7.
[131] Zhao, X.Y., et al., 1alpha,25-dihydroxyvitamin D3 inhibits prostate cancer cell growth by androgen-dependent and androgen-independent mechanisms. *Endocrinology*, 2000. 141(7): p. 2548-56.
[132] Schwartz, G.G., et al., 1 alpha,25-Dihydroxyvitamin D (calcitriol) inhibits the invasiveness of human prostate cancer cells. *Cancer Epidemiol. Biomarkers Prev.*, 1997. 6(9): p. 727-32.
[133] Sung, V. and D. Feldman, 1,25-Dihydroxyvitamin D3 decreases human prostate cancer cell adhesion and migration. *Mol. Cell Endocrinol.*, 2000. 164(1-2): p. 133-43.
[134] Mantell, D.J., et al., 1 alpha,25-dihydroxyvitamin D(3) inhibits angiogenesis in vitro and in vivo. *Circ Res.*, 2000. 87(3): p. 214-20.
[135] Bernardi, R.J., et al., Antiproliferative effects of 1alpha,25-dihydroxyvitamin D(3) and vitamin D analogs on tumor-derived endothelial cells. *Endocrinology*, 2002. 143(7): p. 2508-14.

[136] Krishnan, A.V., et al., Analysis of vitamin D-regulated gene expression in LNCaP human prostate cancer cells using cDNA microarrays. *Prostate,* 2004. 59(3): p. 243-51.
[137] Peehl, D.M., A.V. Krishnan, and D. Feldman, Pathways mediating the growth-inhibitory actions of vitamin D in prostate cancer. *J. Nutr.*, 2003. 133(7 Suppl): p. 2461S-2469S.
[138] Osborn, J.L., et al., Phase II trial of oral 1,25-dihydroxyvitamin D (calcitriol) in hormone refractory prostate cancer. *Urol. Oncol.*, 1995. 1(5): p. 195-8.
[139] Gross, C., et al., Treatment of early recurrent prostate cancer with 1,25-dihydroxyvitamin D3 (calcitriol). *J. Urol.,* 1998. 159(6): p. 2035-9; discussion 2039-40.
[140] Beer, T.M., et al., High-dose weekly oral calcitriol in patients with a rising PSA after prostatectomy or radiation for prostate carcinoma. *Cancer,* 2003. 97(5): p. 1217-24.
[141] Beer, T.M., et al., Pharmacokinetics and tolerability of a single dose of DN-101, a new formulation of calcitriol, in patients with cancer. *Clin. Cancer Res.*, 2005. 11(21): p. 7794-9.
[142] Beer, T.M., et al., Phase I study of weekly DN-101, a new formulation of calcitriol, in patients with cancer. *Cancer Chemother Pharmacol,* 2007. 59(5): p. 581-7.
[143] Beer, T.M., et al., Double-blinded randomized study of high-dose calcitriol plus docetaxel compared with placebo plus docetaxel in androgen-independent prostate cancer: a report from the ASCENT Investigators. *J. Clin. Oncol,* 2007. 25(6): p. 669-74.
[144] Trump, D.L., K.K. Deeb, and C.S. Johnson, Vitamin D: considerations in the continued development as an agent for cancer prevention and therapy. *Cancer J.,* 2010. 16(1): p. 1-9.
[145] Schwartz, G.G., et al., Phase I/II study of 19-nor-1alpha-25-dihydroxyvitamin D2 (paricalcitol) in advanced, androgen-insensitive prostate cancer. *Clin. Cancer Res.*, 2005. 11(24 Pt 1): p. 8680-5.
[146] Liu, G., et al., Phase II study of 1alpha-hydroxyvitamin D(2) in the treatment of advanced androgen-independent prostate cancer. *Clin. Cancer Res.*, 2003. 9(11): p. 4077-83.
[147] Attia, S., et al., Randomized, double-blinded phase II evaluation of docetaxel with or without doxercalciferol in patients with metastatic, androgen-independent prostate cancer. *Clin. Cancer Res.*, 2008. 14(8): p. 2437-43.
[148] Woo, T.C., et al., Pilot study: potential role of vitamin D (Cholecalciferol) in patients with PSA relapse after definitive therapy. *Nutr. Cancer*, 2005. 51(1): p. 32-6.
[149] Krishnan, A.V., D.M. Peehl, and D. Feldman, Vitamin D and Prostate Cancer, in Vitamin D. 2005, Elsevier Academic Press: San Diego. p. 1679-707.
[150] Lips, P., Which circulating level of 25-hydroxyvitamin D is appropriate? *J. Steroid Biochem. Mol. Biol.*, 2004. 89-90(1-5): p. 611-4.
[151] Langlois, K., et al., Vitamin D status of Canadians as measured in the 2007 to 2009 Canadian Health Measures Survey. *Health Rep.*, 2010. 21(1): p. 47-55.

In: Vitamin D Deficiency
Editors: V. Lerner and C. Miodownik
ISBN: 978-1-61470-964-0

Chapter VII

Vitamin D Deficiency in Children and Adolescents

Pisit Pitukcheewanont[1*], Shwu-Fang Lin[2] and Natavut Punyasavatsut[3]
Center of Endocrinology, Diabetes, and Metabolism,
Childrens Hospital Los Angeles, US
[1] Department of Pediatrics, The Keck School of Medicine
of University of Southern California, Los Angeles, California, US
[2] Division of Pediatric Nephrology,
University of Texas Medical Branch, Galveston, Texas, US
[3] Department of Pediatrics, Children's Healthcare
of Atlanta at Scottish Rite, Atlanta, Georgia, US

Abstract

Vitamin D deficiency is quite common among children and adolescents in the United States and worldwide. The high prevalence of vitamin D deficiency during childhood is of major public health concern. Many evidences suggested that vitamin D deficiency may play a significant role in the pathophysiology of other chronic diseases (non-skeletal effect) including autoimmune conditions, cardiovascular diseases, and cancer beyond its skeletal effect (rickets). Early identification, treatment, and prevention of vitamin D deficiency in childhood may have profound health effects throughout the life span. In this chapter, we will discuss the definitions, epidemiology, clinical implications, and treatment of vitamin D deficiency in children and adolescents.

[*] Correspondence and requested reprints: Pisit Pitukcheewanont, MD, Associate Professor of Clinical Pediatrics Department of Pediatrics Childrens Hospital Los Angeles, 4650 Sunset Blvd, Mailstop #61, Los Angeles, Ca 90027, Tel: 323-361-2500, Fax: 323-361 1301 Email: dpisit@chla.usc.edu.

Keywords: Vitamin D, Vitamin D deficiency, Hypovitaminosis D, Bone health, Children, Adolescents, Bone Mineral Density. Skeletal effect, Non-skeletal effect

Abbreviations

25OHD	25-hydroxyvitamin D;
$1,25(OH)_2D$	1,25-dihydroxyvitamin D;
VDR	vitamin D receptor;
Th	T helper;
IU	international unit;
TLR	toll-like receptor;
PTH	parathyroid hormone;
UV	ultraviolet

Introduction

Vitamin D is a fat-soluble vitamin and can be manufactured from two main sources, sun exposure and vitamin D-containing foods. In United States, the main sources of vitamin D are fortified food. Vitamin D comes in two forms: vitamin D2 (Ergocalciferol) and vitamin D3 (Cholecalciferol). Vitamin D3 is the most effective form and more potent than Vitamin D2 for maintaining adequate levels of vitamin D in the body.

Vitamin D, in its active form of Calcitriol, 1,25-dihydroxyvitamin D ($1,25\ (OH)_2D$), acts as a hormone to regulate calcium absorption from the intestine and to regulate levels of calcium and phosphate in the bones. Sunlight is important to skin production of vitamin D, and environmental conditions where sunlight exposure is limited may reduce this source of vitamin D.

Vitamin D helps build strong bones and teeth, strengthen the immune system, maintain joint and muscle comfort, prevent cardiovascular risk and decrease cancer risk in organs such as breast, colon and prostate.

Despite available food sources of vitamin D and the body's ability to self-produce this nutrient from sun exposure, vitamin D deficiency is a worldwide health problem affecting people of all ages. We continue to see low vitamin D levels among the U.S. population, with 70% or more of children having an insufficient vitamin D status [1].

Lack of vitamin D can be associated with bone diseases include osteomalacia (known as rickets in children), caused by a severe and prolonged deficiency of vitamin D and more commonly, osteoporosis, which may arise in part as the result of a sub-optimal state of vitamin D nutrition.

This chapter reviews several aspects of vitamin D biology and metabolism, the physiological roles of vitamin D, and it also defines vitamin D status (vitamin D deficiency vs. insufficiency) based on the published data. This chapter also includes the effect of vitamin D on skeletal and extra-skeletal systems in children and adolescents.

Vitamin D

Vitamin D is a group of fat-soluble secosteroids. Two major physiologically forms are vitamin D2 (ergocalciferol) and vitamin D3 (cholecalciferol) (see figure 1). Vitamin D without a subscript refers to either D_2 or D_3 or both.

Is Vitamin D a Vitamin or a Hormone? Vitamin D is not a vitamin in the strict definition because it can be produced by exposure of the skin to sunlight .As such, animals and humans do not have a dietary requirement for vitamin D when sufficient sunlight is available. However, nutritional vitamin D becomes essential when sunlight is insufficient to meet daily needs. Exposed to sub-optimal levels of sunlight, air pollution, clothes, tall buildings, indoor dwelling, and sunscreens block ultraviolet (UV) light from the sun and these factors all reduce the ability of the skin to synthesize vitamin D.

Vitamin D2 (ergocalciferol) structure   Vitamin D3 (cholecalciferol) structure

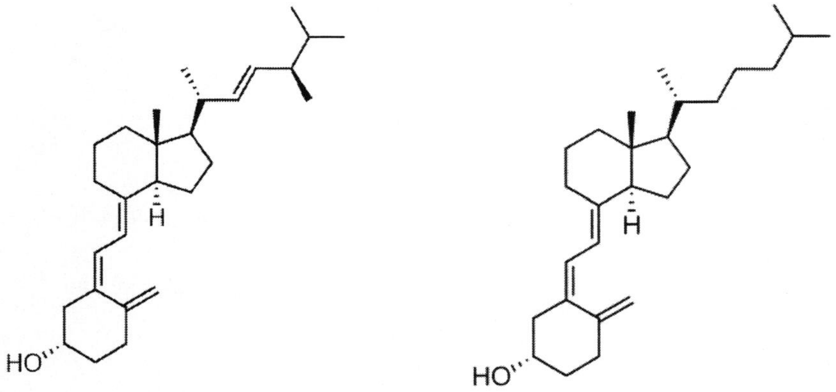

Figure 1. Structures of vitamin D.

The Unit Definition of Vitamin D

The World Health Organization has defined the 'International Unit' (IU) of vitamin D_3 as the activity of 0.025 g of the international standard preparation of crystalline vitamin D_3. One IU of vitamin D_3 equals 0.025g, or 65 pmol. The unit definition of the active metabolite, calcitriol was set to be equivalent in molar terms to that of the parent vitamin D_3. Thus, 1 unit is 65 pmol of calcitriol; as such the unit of calcitriol is much more active than the unit of vitamin D itself. The vitamin D requirements for children or adults have not been precisely defined. Historically, it was defined on the basis of the vitamin D content in a teaspoon of fish oil, a quantity shown to be sufficient to prevent rickets.

Sources of Vitamin D

Sun Exposure

The major source of vitamin D in human and animal is sun exposure. When sunlight exposure is not sufficient, nutritional vitamin D becomes essential.

Nutrition

Children get vitamin D from their diet, dietary supplements and sun exposure. Not many natural foods contain vitamin D. The main natural sources of vitamin D are some fish flesh, fish liver, fish oil and fish liver oil. Other natural sources such as cheese, beef liver and eggs have small amount of Vitamin D. In United States, the main sources of vitamin D are fortified cow milk. Other fortified products include, juices, cereal, bread, yogurt and margarine. Dairy products made from milk, such as cheese and ice cream, are generally not fortified.

Physiology

Synthesis of Vitamin D3

Skin and sunlight:

Solar UVB photons are absorbed by the skin, leading to a chemical reaction that results in the formation of pre-vitamin D_3. Pre-vitamin D_3 is made in the skin when 7-dehydrocholesterol (7-DHC, pro-vitamin D_3) reacts with UVB light at wavelength between 270–300 nm, with peak synthesis occurring between 295-297 nm.

Once formed, pre-vitamin D3 undergoes a thermally induced isomerization over a period of a few hours and is transformed to vitamin D3 (cholecalciferol, inactive).

Vitamin D is transported from skin into the circulation, where it is bound to the vitamin D-binding protein [2].

Although chronic excessive exposure to sunlight increases the risk of non-melanoma skin cancer, the avoidance of all direct sun exposure increases the risk of vitamin D deficiency, which can have serious consequences. The latitude, seasons and time of the day influence vitamin D production. Twenty minutes, three times a week midday sun in low latitudes such as southern CA provides adequate vitamin D stores.

Vitamin D_3 (cholecalciferol, inactive) is synthesized from sun exposure and obtained from nutrition (animals). Vitamin D_2 (ergocalciferol) comes from ingestion of yeasts and plant. Both vitamin D_2 and vitamin D_3 are biologically inert and must undergo two hydroxylations in the liver and kidney for activation respectively.

Liver

Both vitamin D_2 and D_3 are hydroxylated in the liver to 25-hydroxyvitamin D (25OHD) or calcidiol by the enzyme 25-hydroxylase produced by hepatocyte. 25OHD is the major circulating form of vitamin D. The activity of enzyme 25-hydroxylase is not significantly regulated by other hormones or calcium level therefore the level of 25OHD is related to ingestion of vitamin D and sun exposure.

Kidney

Calcidiol, 25OHD is transported to the proximal tubules of the kidneys where it can be hydroxylated by 1α-hydroxylase enzyme to active vitamin D (1,25$(OH)_2$ D) or calcitriol which will have a significant effect on calcium and phosphate homeostasis at the level of gastrointestinal tract, bone and kidney The enzyme 1α-hydroxylase is activated by parathyroid hormone (PTH) and additionally by low calcium or phosphate. Magnesium also plays an important role on regulating PTH secretion and action but not synthesis.

In order to regulate 25OHD and 1,25$(OH)_2$ D, 24-hydroxylase enzyme will hydroxylate both substrates to an inactive form of 24,25$(OH)_2$ D and 1,24,25(OH) D which called calcitroic acid (water –soluble substrate). This metabolite will then be excreted via bile. This 24-OH enzyme is very important to regulate endogenous vitamin D synthesis which will prevent vitamin D intoxication.

Effect of Vitamin D

Calcitriol mediates its biological effects by binding to the vitamin D receptor (VDR), which is principally located in the nuclei of target cells. The vitamin D receptor belongs to the nuclear receptor superfamily of steroid/thyroid hormone receptors, and VDRs are expressed by cells in most organs, including the brain, heart, skin, gonads, prostate, and breast.

VDR activation in the intestine, bone, kidney, and parathyroid gland cells leads to the maintenance of calcium and phosphorus levels in the blood (with the assistance of PTH and calcitonin) and to the maintenance of bone content. Vitamin D is essential to maintain bone health, blood level of calcium and phosphorus. It promotes absorption of calcium and phosphorus in gastrointestinal tract. When dietary calcium is not adequate to maintain blood calcium level, calcitriol increases mobilization of calcium stores by inducing stem cells in the bone marrow to differentiate into osteoclasts.

Definition of Vitamin D status

Vitamin D status is defined by measuring 25OHD concentrations. This serum vitamin D level refers to total combined vitamin D2 and vitamin D3. There is no consensus on the level of serum 25OHD for vitamin D status. Using maximal suppression of PTH by vitamin D, the cut off value for normal plasma 25OHD concentration vary widely but cluster in the 27.5 to 30 ng/mL (67.5 to 75 nmol/L) range [3]. Associations with chronic disease end-points in older adults, e.g. osteoporosis and colorectal cancer as well as associations with linear growth and bone mass in infants, the absence of signs and symptoms of vitamin D deficiency in children are also used to define normal 25OHD concentration [4-6]. In addition, there was considerable variability in the assay used to measure 25OHD concentration.

Vitamin D Insufficiency

Although there is no consensus on the optimal 25OHD concentration for skeletal health, a US expert panel considered a 25OHD concentration of ≥27.5 nmol/L (11 ng/mL) as an indicator of adequate vitamin D status from birth through 18 y and a concentration of ≥30 nmol/L (12 ng/mL) for adults aged 19–50 y [4, 7]. The panel based these values on their associations with linear growth and bone mass in infants, the absence of signs and symptoms of vitamin D deficiency in children, and the relation of 25OHD with PTH concentrations and calcium balance in adults. A UK expert panel considered a plasma on concentration of ≥25 nmol/L (10 ng/mL) as an index of suboptimal vitamin D status [8]. Some [5, 7, 9, 10] suggest that a minimum level of 30 ng/mL (75 nmol/L) is necessary in older adults for overall health and disease prevention but insufficient data are available to support them [8]. This value is higher than the lower end of the reference range, suggesting that the lower end of current reference range is too low.

The report from the Drug and Therapeutics Committee of the Lawson Wilkins Pediatric Endocrine Society has recommended that a serum 25OHD level of >50 nmol/L (20 ng/ mL) is considered as indicative of vitamin D sufficiency and level of 37.5-50.0 nmol/L (15-20 ng/ mL) as vitamin D Insufficiency for children [11].

Vitamin D Deficiency

Similar to vitamin D insufficiency, there is no consistent definitions of vitamin D deficiency. The values range from < 5 ng/mL to <20 ng/dL [12, 13].

The report from the Drug and Therapeutics Committee of the Lawson Wilkins Pediatric Endocrine Society has recommended that a serum 25OHD level of ≤37.5 nmol/L (15 ng/mL) is considered indicative of deficiency and ≤12.5 nmol/L (5 ng/mL) as severe deficiency for children [11].

Severe vitamin D deficiency generally presents as rickets and osteomalacia in children and osteomalacia in adults. However, plasma 25OHD concentration in rickets and osteomalacia ranges from the undetectable to around 8 ng/mL (20 nmol/l) [14].

Prevalence of Vitamin D Insufficiency, Vitamin D Deficiency and Rickets

The prevalence of low vitamin D status depends on the definition, race, season, life cycle, sex, latitude, assay, fortification of vitamin D and state of health. The prevalence is higher in dark skin, winter, elderly female, lack of vitamin D fortification etc.

North America

Neonate

One study [15] consisted of 40 mother-newborn pairs, Neonates were classified as vitamin D deficient (<15 ng/mL), vitamin D insufficient (15-32 ng/mL), or vitamin D sufficient (>32 ng/mL). Among white neonates, 9.7% had vitamin D deficiency, and 56.4% had vitamin D insufficiency. Among black neonates, 45.6% were vitamin D deficient and 46.8% were vitamin D insufficient. The prevalence was higher in white neonate born in spring.

Infants and Older Children

The National Health and Nutrition Examination Survey (NHANES) has included data on serum 25OHD concentrations for persons 12 y or older [4, 16]. National Center for Health Statistics (NCHS) extended the NHANES data collection to include children older than 1 y or older. Using values below the traditional cutoff of <27.5 nmol/L (11 ng/mL), the prevalence was <1%for infants and children aged <11 y, and 5% for adolescents aged 12–19 y. Other studies [17-21] had similar data or higher prevalence when the similar cutoff value compared. The prevalence was 12.4%, and 40% for infant and toddler aged 8-24 months [19].

In North America, there is no current definitive prevalence of rickets estimates available because recent publications have been mainly case reports. Many groups have noted an increased prevalence of rickets in the U.S. [22]. A review of nutritional rickets report among US children <18 y of age published between 1986 and 2003 identified 166 cases of rickets in 22 published studies [23]. From a survey of 2325 Canadian pediatricians, the overall annual incidence rate was 2.9 cases per 100 000. There were 104 confirmed cases of vitamin D deficiency rickets during the study period from July 1, 2002, to June 30, 2004 [24].

Other Countries

Nutritional rickets remains prevalent in many parts of the world [25]. In Europe, Asia and Africa where very few foods are fortified with vitamin D, children would appear to be at especial risk. [10]. Comparing study prevalence estimates can be challenging due to varying definitions of vitamin D deficiency and assay techniques. Many studies provide incomplete data regarding vitamin D deficiency risk factors. Many studies reported prevalence using 25OHD level of ≤ 30 ng/mL vitamin D insufficiency. Estimates suggest that up to 1 billion people around the world may have vitamin insufficiency, if insufficiency is defined as a 25OHD level ≤ 30 ng/mL [19].

In south Asia, Atiq et al. investigated hypovitaminosis D in healthy breast-fed children and nursing mothers at a major teaching hospital in Karachi, Pakistan, and found that 55% of infants and 45% of mothers had very low serum 25OHD levels (<25 nmol/l or 10 ng/ml) [26].

In China, the prevalence of clinical vitamin D and calcium deficiency (plasma 25OHD < 12.5 nmol/L, plasma calcium < 2.25 mmol/L, and muscle spasm at least once per week) was 9.4% in winter [27]. Prevalence of active rickets among rural children in northern China was 3.7 % by using an integrated diagnostic method exploiting clinical signs, X-ray and alkaline phosphatase levels [28].

Possible causes and risk factors for low vitamin D status.

1) Pregnancy and breast feeding
2) Lack of prenatal care in mother
3) Dark skin complexion
4) High altitude, pollution
5) Excessive use of sunscreen
6) Specific religion such as Muslim: covering themselves
7) Obesity
8) Medication such as anticonvulsant, glucocorticoid and anti-rejection agents.
9) Medical condition such as nephrotic syndrome, malabsorbtion and liver failure

Pregnancy and Breast Feeding

Maternal vitamin D status during pregnancy may program skeletal development and body composition in the offspring by influencing the interaction between osteoblasts and adipocytes .

Low maternal serum 25OHD is associated with shorter duration of gestation and, consequently, reduced growth of long bones in newborns. In vitamin D-deficient mothers, maternal PTH is elevated, probably due to increased mineral demands of larger babies. Children of mothers with low vitamin D status during late pregnancy had reduced whole-body bone mineral content, bone area, and areal bone mineral density (BMD) at the age of 9 yr. This suggests that vitamin D has an influence on skeletal programming and the tracking of bone mass lasts throughout childhood.

In the third National Health and Nutrition Examination Survey, 1546 African American women and 1426 white women aged 15–49 y who were not pregnant and who participated (1988–1994) were analyzed. Hypovitaminosis D was defined as a serum 25OHD concentration ≤37.5 nmol/L. The prevalence is high among African American and white women of reproductive age. The prevalence of hypovitaminosis D was 42.4 +/- 3.1% (x +/- SE) among African Americans and 4.2 +/- 0.7% among whites [29].

Neonates born of mothers with low 25OHD levels will also have poor vitamin D status from the start and will be at increased risk of developing hypocalcemic seizures and congenital rickets.

Human breast milk normally contains only small amounts of vitamin D metabolites, including 25OHD, and infants who are breast-fed and do not receive vitamin D supplementation or adequate exposure to sunlight are at high risk of developing vitamin D deficiency or manifesting rickets

Vitamin D in Infancy

The vitamin D status of an infant depends upon the amount of vitamin D transferred from the mother prenatally and upon the amount of vitamin D ingested or produced by the skin during exposure to UV light postnatally.

Increased Skin Pigmentation

Blacks and whites appear to have similar capacities to synthesize vitamin D in the skin but, at usual levels of sun exposure, vitamin D synthesis is less efficient among blacks because of their greater skin pigmentation. Blacks have greater skin melanin pigmentation and, thus, require longer exposures to sunlight to make the same amount of vitamin D3, compared with light-skinned people [30].

Excessive Use of Sunscreen

Sunscreen Study

The use of sunscreen factor 8 excludes 95% of UVB light. It has been suggested that the use of sunscreens to prevent skin cancer may actually put the individual at risk of vitamin D deficiency, which in turn may lead to loss of cortical bone and, ultimately, osteoporotic fractures [11].

For adequate vitamin D synthesis, exposure to the midday sun (between 1000 and 1500 hours) for 10 to 15 minutes in the spring, summer, and fall is considered sufficient for light-skinned people. After this extent of exposure, application of a sunscreen with an SPF of >15 is recommended to prevent damaging effects of chronic excessive exposure to sunlight [11].

Low/Decreased Sun Exposure due to Pollution

Vitamin D Pollution Study

A study compared a group of 9-24 month-old children living in an area of Delhi, India that had high levels of atmospheric pollution with a comparable age-matched group of children living in an area of Delhi that had less pollution.

Mean serum 25OHD levels, the biomarker for vitamin D, were compared and it was found that children living in an area of high air pollution had 25OHD levels significantly lower than those living in areas of less pollution [31].

Over Clothing

Vitamin D deficiency rickets were reported more in Muslim population [32].

The Muslim women wear clothes which apart from face and hands cover all other parts of their bodies. Even if they go out, opportunity to expose their bodies in sunlight is not available in the all encompassing "Burqa" (a head to toe covering which only has small openings for the eyes).

HIV Positive Patients

Although subjects with HIV infection are at increased risk of osteopenia and osteoporosis, a cross-sectional study of members of the Reaching for Excellence in Adolescent Health (REACH) cohort concluded that HIV infection did not influence vitamin D status. The subjects were aged 14-23 yr; 74% were female, and 72% were black. Mean plasma 25OHD did not differ significantly (P = 0.62) between the HIV-positive (20.3 +/- 1.1 nmol/L; n = 238) and HIV-negative (19.3 +/- 1.7 nmol/L; n = 121) subjects [33].

Decreased Bioavailability, Decreased Synthesis and Increased Metabolism of 25OHD

Obesity

Interpreting data on 25OHD concentrations for obese and overweight persons is particularly challenging. The NHANES showed lower circulating concentrations of 25OHD among young adult obese non-Hispanic white women than their leaner counterparts [23, 34]. Differences in physical activity partially explained these differences, but the relations appeared to be weaker among non-Hispanic blacks than non-Hispanic whites. Some of these differences might be due to physiologic factors. Obese persons had lower circulating 25OHD concentrations than did leaner persons after supplementation with vitamin D2 and after exposure to UV radiation [32]. However, overweight and obese persons in NHANES also reported lower use of multivitamin-multimineral supplements and vitamin D–containing dietary supplements than did leaner persons of the same age or sex group [35, 36]; these results suggest that low dietary exposures could also contribute to the lower 25OHD concentrations in overweight and obese people. The 2007 UK advisory committee report cited a need to better understand the effects of adiposity on circulating 25OHD concentrations and the implications of the relation between adiposity and 25OHD concentrations for vitamin D requirements [37].

A recent study in NY children and adolescent, 55.2% of patients obese children had vitamin D levels <20 ng/ml with equal gender distribution. Vitamin D insufficiency was associated with increased age, BMI, and SBP, and decreased HDL-C [28].

Malabsorption

Reduction in fat absorption in conditions such as cystic fibrosis, celiac disease, Whipple's disease, Crohn's disease, bypass surgery, medications reducing cholesterol absorption, and Type I Diabetes Mellitus (T1DM) can result decreased vitamin D absorption.

A study is based on matching by age, gender and ethnicity of 170 T1DM children with those of 170 controls healthy subjects below 16 years. The result revealed that vitamin D deficiency was considerably higher in T1DM children (90.6%) compared to non-diabetic children (85.3%) ($p = 0.009$) [38].

Increased Catabolism

It is well recognized that long-term therapy with some antiepileptic drugs, glucocorticoids, and antirejection medication-binding to the steroid and xenobiotic receptor or the preagnane X receptor can cause osteomalacia or increased vitamin D requirement [10, 39]. 1,25(OH)2D3 is catabolized by CYP24 (also known as 25-hydroxyvitamin D 24-hydroxylase) in the kidney and CYP3A4-dependent 23- and 24-hydroxylations in the liver and small intestine [40]. A study suggested that activation of xenobiotic receptor by some drugs induced CYP3A4 expression in liver and intestine, which promotes metabolism of 1,25(OH)2D3 [41].

Urinary Loss

Patient with Nephrotic syndrome has increased loss of 25OHD bound to vitamin D-binding protein in urine.

Decreased Synthesis

Both vitamin D_2 and D_3 are hydroxylated in the liver to 25OHD or calcidiol by the enzyme 25-hydroxylase produced by hepatocyte. Liver dysfunction result decreased synthesis of 25OHD.

Skeletal Effect of Vitamin D

One of the most important roles of vitamin D is to maintain skeletal calcium balance by promoting calcium absorption in the intestines, maintaining calcium and phosphate levels for bone formation, and allowing proper functioning of PTH.

Hypovitaminosis D causes impaired longitudinal bone growth. The cup-shaped metaphysis, widening and disorganization of bone structure result from compensatory proliferation of peripheral growth plate cartilage cells. This type of 'epiphyseal dysplasia' is defined as 'rickets' a constitutional disease of childhood [42].

The gastrointestinal symptoms and signs precede the manifestation of poor growth and bone changes. The appetite is diminished, and there is frequent vomiting, together with diarrhea. Other symptoms in the early stages are bone pain and sweating of the head and upper parts of the body, particularly during sleep.

Gradually the changes in the shape of the bones become visible, at first chiefly noticed at the ends of the long bones, as in those of the arm, causing enlargements at the wrists, or in the ribs (rachitic rosary). The bones tend to become distorted, both by the action of the muscles and by the superincumbent weight of the body. Lower extremities appear "bowlegged" or "in-kneed". The trunk of the body likewise shows various alterations and deformities owing to curvatures of the spine, the flattening of the lateral curves of the ribs, and the projection forwards of the sternum. The pelvis distortion may reduce its capacity to a degree that in the female may afterwards lead to serious difficulties in parturition. The head of the child with severe rickets is large-looking in its upper part, the individual bones of the cranium sometimes remaining long ununited, while the face is small and ill-developed, and the teeth appear late and fall out or decay early [42] .

Classification of Rickets

Rickets can be secondary to different etiologies. Among them, nutritional, genetic, drug induced, and prematurity are the most common. John Pettifor [43, 44] classified rickets in ''calciopenic'' (secondary to alterations of vitamin D metabolism or dietary calcium deficiency), ''phosphopenic'' (caused by dietary phosphate deficiency, impaired intestinal absorption of phosphate, increased renal phosphate loss, etc.), and ''inhibition of mineralization'' (e.g., hereditary hypophosphatasia, aluminum and fluoride toxicity, and first-generation bisphosphonates).

Osteomalacia

It usually occurs in adolescents when epiphyseal plates had been closed. As vitamin D deficiency progresses, the parathyroid glands are maximally stimulated, causing secondary hyperparathyroidism. Osteomalacia, the bone disease in vitamin D deficiency, results from inadequate mineralization of bone matrix with increased bone mass .It is to be distinguished from osteoporosis where bone mass is decreased, from hypophosphatemic osteopenia of premature infants, and from renal osteodystrophy, which is partly due to calcitriol renal deficiency, but also due to hyperphosphatemic hyperparathyroidism.

Extra- Skeletal Effect of Vitamin D

Vitamin D is not just for bone anymore. It has effect of cell differentiation and proliferation not associated with bone and calcium metabolisms. The vitamin D binding receptor is not only expressed in tissues involved in calcium homeostasis but also found in more than 36 other tissue types. Directly or indirectly, $1,25(OH)_2$ D controls more than 200 genes, including genes responsible for the regulation of cellular proliferation, differentiation, apoptosis, and angiogenesis [10]. Vitamin D has more recently been implicated in a number of additional pathological processes .These processes include cancer, multiple sclerosis, psoriasis and the inflammatory response, supporting a role for vitamin D in delineating healthy trajectories of aging.

Cardiovascular System

Meta-analysis provides a complete picture of the potentially beneficial role that high levels of 25OHD may provide on cardio-metabolic health. The association was significant across all cardio-metabolic disease outcomes and study designs, in 28 studies including 99,745 participants across a variety of ethnic groups and in both men and women [45]. Their findings suggest that high levels of vitamin D, among adult populations, are associated with a substantial decrease in cardiovascular disease, type 2 diabetes (T2DM) and metabolic syndrome. Interventions targeting a positive modification of vitamin D deficiency in adult and elderly populations could substantially contribute to halting the current epidemics of cardiometabolic disorders. Further controlled trials are required to evaluate the causal association between vitamin D levels and cardiometabolic disorders as well as the benefit of vitamin D supplementation in the reduction of cardiometabolic disease.

Diabetes

$1,25(OH)_2$ D stimulates insulin secretion, presumably by regulating calcium flux, although the mechanism is not well defined. Pittas et al. [46] recently published a meta-analysis of studies demonstrating a link between vitamin D deficiency and T2DM.

In particular, in non-blacks, the relative risk (RR) of T2 DM was 0.36 in those with the highest 25OHD levels compared to those with the lowest levels. In a recent Finnish trial [47] with a 22-year follow up of 7503 subjects free of diabetes at the beginning of the trial, subjects with the highest 25OHD levels at the start of the trial had a RR of 0.6 for developing DM compared to those with the lowest 25OHD levels. Long-term randomized controlled trials with vitamin D supplementation are needed to confirm these mostly observational cross-sectional and case-control studies.

Cancer

Vitamin D's possible role in the prevention of some types of cancer is one of the most important areas of research involving vitamin D. People living at higher latitudes are at increased risk for Hodgkin's lymphoma as well as colon, pancreatic, prostate, ovarian, breast, and other cancers [10]. 1,25$(OH)_2$ D is involved, via its nuclear vitamin D receptor (VDR), in the regulation of cell differentiation, cell growth, apoptosis (cell death) and various cellular mechanisms that play a role in cancer development. 1,25$(OH)_2$ D has a role in inducing apoptosis and inhibiting angiogenesis once a cell becomes malignant, therefore reducing the ability of the malignant cell to survive. Colon, prostate and mammary cells have demonstrated the ability to extra-renally synthesize 1,25$(OH)_2$ D, which may play a role in modulating cell proliferation and apoptosis at the local level. The main types of cancer that vitamin D has been linked to are colorectal, breast and prostate; however, links with other types of cancer such as lung, ovarian and endometrial have also been suggested [48].

Immune System

The link between vitamin D deficiency and susceptibility to infection has been suggested for longer than a century, with the early observation that children with nutritional rickets were more likely to experience infections of the respiratory system, leading to the coining of the phrase "rachitic lung" [49]. VDRs are found in activated dendritic cells, macrophages and lymphocytes. Two forms of immunity exist; adaptive and innate. Each are regulated by 1,25$(OH)_2$ D [50]. 1,25$(OH)_2$ D is a potent immunomodulator. Several studies demonstrate a likely connection among vitamin D repletion, susceptibility to infection, and clinical outcomes in a variety of infectious processes [51]. Current evidence supports further research into adjunctive vitamin D therapy for Tuberculosis, Influenza and viral upper respiratory tract infection.

Adaptive Immunity

Antigen presenting cells, primarily dendritic cells, macrophages and some other cells such as keratinocytes, when activated induce the proliferation and differentiation of T cells (CD 4and CD8) along different pathways depending on a variety of conditions including cell context and type of antigen activating the system. The dendritic cell can stimulate CD 4cell to differentiate into one of four different types of T helper (Th) cells. 1,25$(OH)_2$ D influences this process by inhibiting the development of Th1 and Th17 cells, while promoting that of Th 2and Treg cells [50].

Innate Immunity

Several of activated toll-like receptors (TLRs) induce VDR and CYP27B1. With adequate substrate (25OHD), this results in 1,25$(OH)_2$ D production within the cell .In turn, 1,25$(OH)_2$D binds to the VDR to induce antimicrobial peptides such as cathelicidin capable of killing the invading organism .Monocytes and macrophages exposed to a lipopolysaccharide or to Mycobacterium tuberculosis up-regulate the vitamin D receptor gene and the 25-hydroxyvitamin D1α hydroxylase gene. Increased production of 1,25$(OH)_2$ D results in synthesis of cathelecidin, which destroys M. tuberculosis as well as other infectious agents. When serum levels of 25OHD fall below 20 ng per milliliter (50 nmol per liter), the monocyte or macrophage is prevented from initiating this innate immune response, which may explain why black Americans, who are often vitamin D–deficient, are more prone to contracting tuberculosis than are whites, and tend to have a more aggressive form of the disease [10, 52]. The innate immune response is also critical for activating the adaptive immune response, but the role of 1,25$(OH)_2$ D in this process has received limited study.

Autoimmune Disease

Multiple Scleriosis (MS)

Vitamin D is one of the most attractive candidates among various environmental factors suggested to be involved in the development of the disease. Supplement with vitamin D may reduce the risk of conversion from a first clinical event suggestive of MS to clinical definite MS, as well as reduce the relapse rate among patients with relapsing remitting MS [53].

Psoriasis

Previously psoriasis had been viewed as primarily a disease of hyperproliferation, more recently it has come to be regarded as an immune-mediated disease [54]. Topical vitamin D agents have been developed as a newer therapeutic option for use in place of, or in addition to, topical corticosteroids. These agents act to inhibit keratinocyte proliferation, normalize differentiation and modulate the activity of immune cells with minimal effect on serum calcium homeostasis.

Calcipotriene is the most widely used member of this class, and is one of the most frequently prescribed topical agents for psoriasis. Although evidence suggests that it is approximately as effective as low-to-medium potency corticosteroids, it is associated with cutaneous irritation, especially when used in sensitive areas. Calcitriol ointment is a new option for topical therapy and is the only vitamin D 3ointment available for use in the U.S . and contains the naturally occurring active form of vitamin D_3 that is associated with a relatively low rate of side effects .

Schizophrenia and Depression

Vitamin D deficiency has been linked to an increased incidence of schizophrenia and depressions. Maintaining vitamin D sufficiency in utero and during early life, to satisfy the vitamin D receptor transcriptional activity in the brain, may be important for brain development as well as for maintenance of mental function [10].

Treatment

Vitamin D

Vitamins D2 and D3 are generally considered to be equivalent in humans. However, a study of 20 healthy male volunteers showed longer sustained level in Vitamin D3. The single dose of 50,000 IU both calciferols produced similar rises in serum concentration of the administered vitamin, but 25OHD continued to rise in the vitamin D3 treated subjects, peaking at 14 d, whereas serum 25OHD fell rapidly in the vitamin D2-treated subjects and was not different from baseline at 14 d [55].

Conventional Dose

Infant and Children

Dosing regimens for nutritional deficiency are similar to those used for vitamin D deficient rickets. Our recommendation is to use doses of 1000 IU/day for infants < 1 month old, 1000 to 5000 IU/day for infants 1 to 12 months old, and 5000 -15,000 IU/day for children >12 months old [56]. Short term vitamin D2 2,000 IU daily, vitamin D2 50,000 IU weekly, or vitamin D3 2,000 IU daily yield equivalent outcomes in the treatment of hypovitaminosis D among young children [57]. With therapy, radiological evidence of healing is observed in 2 to 4 weeks, after which the dose of vitamin D can be reduced to 400 IU/day.

Stoss (“stoss” therapy, from the German stossen meaning “to push”),

Lack of compliance is an important cause of lack of response, and an option after the first month of life is to administer high doses of vitamin D in a single administration (100,000–600,000 IU IM or PO over 1–5 days) [34, 37, 56] followed by maintenance dosing. High-dose vitamin D may need to be intermittently repeated (usually every 3 -6months) if poor compliance persists with maintenance dosing. Preparations of ergocalciferol solution in propylene glycol should not be used for the treatment of rickets with high dosages because of possible propylene intoxication. For infants, soaking a 50 000-IU capsule in a small amount of water to soften it or crushing a 25,000 IU or 50,000-IU vitamin D tablet [11, 34] before administration in blended baby food can be used.

Calcium

Hypocalcemia should be treated with calcium supplements. In addition to calcium supplements, calcitriol may be necessary in doses of 0.02 -0.08 mcg/kg per day in 2 to 3 divided doses until calcium levels normalize. Even for children who are not hypocalcemic, calcium supplements are important for avoiding subsequent hypocalcemia from "hungry-bone" syndrome, particularly with stoss therapy.

Prophylaxis/Vitamin D Supplement

Sufficient vitamin D status in early life is essential for bone health. Supplementation with vitamin D should therefore be recommended for known risk groups for development of rickets, such as breast-fed infants, children with milk intake less than 1 L per day, infants and children with fat malabsorption, and dark-skinned children from both sunny and non-sunny countries who avoid sun exposure or live in areas with severe air pollution. Children with some liver and kidney diseases may need active vitamin D supplement.

There is no recommended daily allowance (RDA) for vitamin D. Recommendations for vitamin D intake are actually referred to as ''adequate intake'' (AI). AI is established when evidence is insufficient to develop an RDA and is set at a level assumed to ensure nutritional adequacy.

Intake reference values for vitamin D and other nutrients are provided in the Dietary Reference Intakes (DRIs) developed by the Food and Nutrition Board (FNB) at the Institute of Medicine of The National Academies (formerly National Academy of Sciences) [58]. The current DRIs for calcium and vitamin D was released on 11/30/2010 (Table 1).

Intake of vitamin D-containing food products should also be retained. Eating oily fish such as salmon and mackerel three or four times weekly is usually adequate to meet the vitamin D requirement in children.

In 2003, the American Academy of Pediatrics (AAP) recommended a vitamin D supplement 200 IU per day for (1) breastfed infants (2) non-breastfed infants and children who do not consume >500 mL of vitamin D–fortified beverages. However, despite the previous guidelines for vitamin D supplementation, rickets continues to be reported. In 2007 and 2008, Pediatric Endocrine Society (Lawson Wilkin Pediatric Endocrinology Society) and AAP respectively, recommended vitamin D intake that exceed AI of FNB. They recommended that all breastfed infants, and non-breastfed infants and children who do not ingest at least 1 L of vitamin D–fortified milk per day, receive 400 IU vitamin D per day as a supplement [11].

Table 1. Dietary Reference Intakes for Calcium and Vitamin D

	Calcium			Vitamin D		
Life Stage Group	**Estimated Average Requirment (mg/day)**	**Recommended Dietary Allowance (mg/day)**	**Upper Level Intake (mg/day)**	**Estimatee Average Requirment (IU/day)**	**Recommended Dietary Allowwance (IU/day)**	**Upper Level Intake (IU/day)**
Infant 0 to 6 months	*	*	1,000	**	**	1,000
Infants 6 to 12 months	*	*	1,500	**	**	1,500
1-3 years old	500	700	2,500	400	600	2,500
4-8 years old	800	1,000	2,500	400	600	3,000
9-13 years old	1,100	1,300	3,000	400	600	4,000
14-18 years old	1,100	1,300	3,000	400	600	4,000
19-30 years old	800	1,000	2,500	400	600	4,000
31-50 years old	800	1,000	2,500	400	600	4,000
51-70 year old males	800	1,000	2,000	400	600	4,000
51-70 year old females	1,000	1,200	2,000	400	600	4,000
>70 years old	1,000	1,200	2,000	400	800	4,000
14-18 years old, pregnant/lactating	1,100	1,300	3,000	400	600	4,000
19-50 years old, pregnant /lactating	800	1,000	2,500	400	600	4,000

*For infants, Adequate Intake is 200 mg/day for 0 to 6 months of age and 260 mg/day for 6 to 12 months of age.

**For infants. Adequate Intake is 400 IU/day for 0 to 6 months of age and 400 IU/day for 6-12 months of age.

The table is adapted from Food and Nutrition Board at the Institute of Medicine.

References

[1] U.S. National Center for Health Statistics. Fat-Soluble Vitamins and Micronutrients: Vitamin DNational Report on Biochemical Indicators of Diet and Nutrition in the U.S. Population 1999–2002.

[2] Favus MJ, American Society for Bone and Mineral Research. Primer on the metabolic bone diseases and disorders of mineral metabolism. 4st ed. [Kelseyville, Calif.]: American Society for Bone and Mineral Research; 1999.

[3] Durazo-Arvizu RA, Dawson-Hughes B, Sempos CT, Yetley EA, Looker AC, Cao G, et al. Three-phase model harmonizes estimates of the maximal suppression of parathyroid hormone by 25-hydroxyvitamin D in persons 65 years of age and older. *J. Nutr.* Mar;140(3):595-9.

[4] Yetley EA. Assessing the vitamin D status of the US population. *Am. J. Clin. Nutr.* 2008 Aug;88(2):558S-64S.

[5] Dawson-Hughes B, Heaney RP, Holick MF, Lips P, Meunier PJ, Vieth R. Estimates of optimal vitamin D status. *Osteoporos Int.* 2005 Jul;16(7):713-6.

[6] Bischoff-Ferrari HA, Giovannucci E, Willett WC, Dietrich T, Dawson-Hughes B. Estimation of optimal serum concentrations of 25-hydroxyvitamin D for multiple health outcomes. *Am. J. Clin. Nutr.* 2006 Jul;84(1):18-28.

[7] U.S. Department of Agriculture. National Nutrient Database for Standard Reference release 20; 2007.

[8] Scientific Advisory Committee on Nutrition. Update on Vitamin D. Position Statement by the Scientific Advisory Committee on Nutrition. London: The Stationery Office; 2007.

[9] Vieth R. What is the optimal vitamin D status for health? *Prog. Biophys. Mol. Biol.* 2006 Sep;92(1):26-32.

[10] Holick MF. Vitamin D deficiency. *N. Engl. J. Med.* 2007 Jul 19;357(3):266-81.

[11] Misra M, Pacaud D, Petryk A, Collett-Solberg PF, Kappy M. Vitamin D deficiency in children and its management: review of current knowledge and recommendations. *Pediatrics*. 2008 Aug;122(2):398-417.

[12] Rovner AJ, O'Brien KO. Hypovitaminosis D among healthy children in the United States: a review of the current evidence. *Arch. Pediatr. Adolesc. Med.* 2008 Jun;162(6):513-9.

[13] Orwoll E, Nielson CM, Marshall LM, Lambert L, Holton KF, Hoffman AR, et al. Vitamin D deficiency in older men. *J. Clin. Endocrinol. Metab.* 2009 Apr;94(4):1214-22.

[14] Department of Health. Nutrition and Bone Health: with particular reference to calcium and vitamin D no. 49. London: The Stationary Office; 1998.

[15] Lee JM, Smith JR, Philipp BL, Chen TC, Mathieu J, Holick MF. Vitamin D deficiency in a healthy group of mothers and newborn infants. *Clin. Pediatr.* (Phila). 2007 Jan;46(1):42-4.

[16] Shah M, Salhab N, Patterson D, Seikaly MG. Nutritional rickets still afflict children in north Texas. *Tex. Med.* 2000 Jun;96(6):64-8.

[17] Sullivan SS, Rosen CJ, Halteman WA, Chen TC, Holick MF. Adolescent girls in Maine are at risk for vitamin D insufficiency. *J. Am. Diet Assoc.* 2005 Jun;105(6):971-4.

[18] El-Hajj Fuleihan G, Nabulsi M, Choucair M, Salamoun M, Hajj Shahine C, Kizirian A, et al. Hypovitaminosis D in healthy schoolchildren. *Pediatrics*. 2001 Apr;107(4):E53.
[19] Gordon CM, Feldman HA, Sinclair L, Williams AL, Kleinman PK, Perez-Rossello J, et al. Prevalence of vitamin D deficiency among healthy infants and toddlers. *Arch. Pediatr. Adolesc. Med.* 2008 Jun;162(6):505-12.
[20] Liang L, Chantry C, Styne DM, Stephensen CB. Prevalence and risk factors for vitamin D deficiency among healthy infants and young children in Sacramento, California. *Eur. J. Pediatr*. 2010 Jun 8;169(11):1337-44.
[21] Gordon CM, DePeter KC, Feldman HA, Grace E, Emans SJ. Prevalence of vitamin D deficiency among healthy adolescents. *Arch Pediatr Adolesc Med.* 2004 Jun;158(6):531-7.
[22] Kreiter SR, Schwartz RP, Kirkman HN, Jr., Charlton PA, Calikoglu AS, Davenport ML. Nutritional rickets in African American breast-fed infants. *J Pediatr*. 2000 Aug;137(2):153-7.
[23] Weisberg P, Scanlon KS, Li R, Cogswell ME. Nutritional rickets among children in the United States: review of cases reported between 1986 and 2003. *Am. J. Clin. Nutr*. 2004 Dec;80(6 Suppl):1697S-705S.
[24] Ward LM, Gaboury I, Ladhani M, Zlotkin S. Vitamin D-deficiency rickets among children in Canada. *Cmaj*. 2007 Jul 17;177(2):161-6.
[25] Bhattacharyya AK. Nutritional rickets in the tropics. *World Rev Nutr Diet.* 1992;67:140-97.
[26] Atiq M, Suria A, Nizami SQ, Ahmed I. Vitamin D status of breastfed Pakistani infants. *Acta Paediatr*. 1998 Jul;87(7):737-40.
[27] Du X, Greenfield H, Fraser DR, Ge K, Trube A, Wang Y. Vitamin D deficiency and associated factors in adolescent girls in Beijing. *Am. J. Clin. Nutr*. 2001 Oct;74(4):494-500.
[28] Smotkin-Tangorra M, Purushothaman R, Gupta A, Nejati G, Anhalt H, Ten S. Prevalence of vitamin D insufficiency in obese children and adolescents. *J Pediatr Endocrinol Metab*. 2007 Jul;20(7):817-23.
[29] Nesby-O'Dell S, Scanlon KS, Cogswell ME, Gillespie C, Hollis BW, Looker AC, et al. Hypovitaminosis D prevalence and determinants among African American and white women of reproductive age: third National Health and Nutrition Examination Survey, 1988-1994. *Am. J. Clin. Nutr*. 2002 Jul;76(1):187-92.
[30] Matsuoka LY, Ide L, Wortsman J, MacLaughlin JA, Holick MF. Sunscreens suppress cutaneous vitamin D3 synthesis. *J. Clin. Endocrinol. Metab*. 1987 Jun;64(6):1165-8.
[31] Agarwal KS, Mughal MZ, Upadhyay P, Berry JL, Mawer EB, Puliyel JM. The impact of atmospheric pollution on vitamin D status of infants and toddlers in Delhi, India. *Arch Dis Child*. 2002 Aug;87(2):111-3.
[32] Bachrach S, Fisher J, Parks JS. An outbreak of vitamin D deficiency rickets in a susceptible population. *Pediatrics*. 1979 Dec;64(6):871-7.
[33] Stephensen CB, Marquis GS, Kruzich LA, Douglas SD, Aldrovandi GM, Wilson CM. Vitamin D status in adolescents and young adults with HIV infection. *Am. J. Clin. Nutr*. 2006 May;83(5):1135-41.
[34] Hochberg Z, Bereket A, Davenport M, Delemarre-Van de Waal HA, De Schepper J, Levine MA, et al. Consensus development for the supplementation of vitamin D in childhood and adolescence. *Horm Res*. 2002;58(1):39-51.

[35] Bowden SA, Robinson RF, Carr R, Mahan JD. Prevalence of vitamin D deficiency and insufficiency in children with osteopenia or osteoporosis referred to a pediatric metabolic bone clinic. *Pediatrics.* 2008 Jun;121(6):e1585-90.

[36] Isaia G, Giorgino R, Rini GB, Bevilacqua M, Maugeri D, Adami S. Prevalence of hypovitaminosis D in elderly women in Italy: clinical consequences and risk factors. *Osteoporos Int.* 2003 Jul;14(7):577-82.

[37] Shah BR, Finberg L. Single-day therapy for nutritional vitamin D-deficiency rickets: a preferred method. *J Pediatr.* 1994 Sep;125(3):487-90.

[38] Bener A, Alsaied A, Al-Ali M, Al-Kubaisi A, Basha B, Abraham A, et al. High prevalence of vitamin D deficiency in type 1 diabetes mellitus and healthy children. *Acta Diabetol.* 2009 Sep;46(3):183-9.

[39] Pack AM, Morrell MJ. Epilepsy and bone health in adults. *Epilepsy Behav.* 2004 Feb;5 Suppl 2:S24-9.

[40] Xu Y, Hashizume T, Shuhart MC, Davis CL, Nelson WL, Sakaki T, et al. Intestinal and hepatic CYP3A4 catalyze hydroxylation of 1alpha,25-dihydroxyvitamin D(3): implications for drug-induced osteomalacia. *Mol Pharmacol.* 2006 Jan;69(1):56-65.

[41] Zhou C, Assem M, Tay JC, Watkins PB, Blumberg B, Schuetz EG, et al. Steroid and xenobiotic receptor and vitamin D receptor crosstalk mediates CYP24 expression and drug-induced osteomalacia. *J Clin Invest.* 2006 Jun;116(6):1703-12.

[42] Hochberg Z. Rickets--past and present. Introduction. *Endocr Dev.* 2003;6:1-13.

[43] Lehtonen-Veromaa M, Mottonen T, Irjala K, Karkkainen M, Lamberg-Allardt C, Hakola P, et al. Vitamin D intake is low and hypovitaminosis D common in healthy 9- to 15-year-old Finnish girls. *Eur. J. Clin Nutr.* 1999 Sep;53(9):746-51.

[44] Daniels ED, Pettifor JM, Moodley GP. Serum osteocalcin has limited usefulness as a diagnostic marker for rickets. *Eur. J. Pediatr.* 2000 Oct;159(10):730-3.

[45] Parker J, Hashmi O, Dutton D, Mavrodaris A, Stranges S, Kandala NB, et al. Levels of vitamin D and cardiometabolic disorders: systematic review and meta-analysis. *Maturitas.* Mar;65(3):225-36.

[46] Pittas AG, Lau J, Hu FB, Dawson-Hughes B. The role of vitamin D and calcium in type 2 diabetes. A systematic review and meta-analysis. *J. Clin. Endocrinol. Metab.* 2007 Jun;92(6):2017-29.

[47] Mattila C, Knekt P, Mannisto S, Rissanen H, Laaksonen MA, Montonen J, et al. Serum 25-hydroxyvitamin D concentration and subsequent risk of type 2 diabetes. *Diabetes Care.* 2007 Oct;30(10):2569-70.

[48] Borradale D, Kimlin M. Vitamin D in health and disease: an insight into traditional functions and new roles for the 'sunshine vitamin'. *Nutr. Res. Rev.* 2009 Dec;22(2):118-36.

[49] Khajavi A, Amirhakimi GH. The rachitic lung. Pulmonary findings in 30 infants and children with malnutritional rickets. *Clin. Pediatr.* (Phila). 1977 Jan;16(1):36-8.

[50] Bikle DD. Vitamin D: newly discovered actions require reconsideration of physiologic requirements. *Trends Endocrinol. Metab.* Jun;21(6):375-84.

[51] Yamshchikov AV, Desai NS, Blumberg HM, Ziegler TR, Tangpricha V. Vitamin D for treatment and prevention of infectious diseases: a systematic review of randomized controlled trials. *Endocr. Pract.* 2009 Jul-Aug;15(5):438-49.

[52] Penna G, Roncari A, Amuchastegui S, Daniel KC, Berti E, Colonna M, et al. Expression of the inhibitory receptor ILT3 on dendritic cells is dispensable for

induction of CD4+Foxp3+ regulatory T cells by 1,25-dihydroxyvitamin D3. *Blood.* 2005 Nov 15;106(10):3490-7.

[53] Myhr KM. Vitamin D treatment in multiple sclerosis. *J. Neurol. Sci.* 2009 Nov 15;286(1-2):104-8.

[54] Nickoloff BJ, Nestle FO. Recent insights into the immunopathogenesis of psoriasis provide new therapeutic opportunities. *J. Clin. Invest.* 2004 Jun;113(12):1664-75.

[55] Armas LA, Hollis BW, Heaney RP. Vitamin D2 is much less effective than vitamin D3 in humans. *J. Clin. Endocrinol. Metab.* 2004 Nov;89(11):5387-91.

[56] Lifshitz F. Pediatric endocrinology. 5th ed. New York: Informa Healthcare; 2007.

[57] Gordon CM, Williams AL, Feldman HA, May J, Sinclair L, Vasquez A, et al. Treatment of hypovitaminosis D in infants and toddlers. *J. Clin. Endocrinol. Metab.* 2008 Jul;93(7):2716-21.

[58] Institute of Medicine of the National Academies. Dietary Reference Intakes for Calcium and Vitamin D: National Academies of sciences; 2010.

In: Vitamin D Deficiency
Editors: V. Lerner and C. Miodownik
ISBN: 978-1-61470-964-0

Chapter VIII

Vitamin D in the Elderly

Tzvi Dwolatzky*
Department of Geriatrics and Memory Clinic, Mental Health Center
Faculty of Health Sciences, Ben-Gurion University of the Negev, Beersheva, Israel

Abstract

Prevalence studies have demonstrated that vitamin D deficiency is widespread among the older population worldwide. While the effects of inadequate levels of vitamin D on calcium metabolism and the development of osteoporosis are well known among health care providers, there is mounting evidence for other consequences of a lack of this vitamin on the health of the elderly. Studies have shown that insufficient levels of vitamin D are associated with functional disability and falls at an advanced age. Vitamin D insufficiency is correlated with the development of cancer, especially of the colon, prostate, breast and lymphoma. Further, lower levels of vitamin D are also associated with the development of cognitive changes, cardiovascular disease and mortality. In this chapter we will discuss the prevalence of vitamin D insufficiency in the elderly, describe the negative effects of a lack of this vitamin on the health of older people, and relate to the possible beneficial effects of vitamin D supplementation in the older population.

Keywords: Vitamin D, elderly, falls, function, cognition, supplementation

Abbreviations

UVB	ultraviolet B
PTH	parathyroid hormone

* Address for correspondence: Tzvi Dwolatzky, M.D., MBBCh. Senior Lecturer, Faculty of Health Sciences, Ben Gurion University of the Negev & Director, Department of Geriatrics and Memory Clinic, Be'er Sheva Mental Health Center. Mailing address: Be'er Sheva Mental Health Center, PO Box 4600, Be'er Sheva 84170, Israel. Tel: 08-6401520 Fax: 08-6401462. E-mail: tzvidov@bgu.ac.il.

WHI	Women's Health Initiative
VDR	vitamin D receptor
CRP	C-reactive protein

Vitamin D Metabolism in the Elderly

As people age the degree of exposure to the sun often decreases due to changes in lifestyle and daily activities. It is common for older people to be more particular about dressing warmly and wearing clothes that cover most of their bodies.

Old people are more likely to spend more of their daytime hours indoors and are less likely to engage in outdoor activities. Dietary vitamin D intake, mainly from fish liver oils and fortified cow's milk, is also limited. However, more important than these factors is that the production of vitamin D by the exposure of the skin to ultraviolet B (UVB) light decreases with age, especially after the age of 70 years. This decline in skin synthesis of vitamin D is due both to atrophic changes as a result of aging of the skin, and a decrease in the amount of its precursor. The age-associated decrease in renal function results in a diminished production by the kidneys of $1,25(OH)_2D$, the most metabolically active form of vitamin D.

Also, since vitamin D is fat-soluble, the progressive loss in mean body mass and relative increase in fat associated with advancing age, results in a greater distribution of this vitamin in body fat with age, and this may increase vitamin D requirements in older people.

Prevalence and Definitions

Vitamin D insufficiency and overt deficiency is common with advancing age, especially in the housebound or institutionalized elderly. There are clearly differences in prevalence depending on the climate, on the population studied, and on lifestyle and cultural differences. The reported prevalence of vitamin D deficiency depends on the level of serum 25-OH vitamin D used to define the normal range. Estimating the optimal concentrations of 25-OH vitamin D, a survey in the USA found that more than 90% of older white adults had concentrations of 36 ng/ml or less [1]. Normal values can be determined either using such population-based studies, or by the physiological response where parathyroid hormone (PTH) begins to rise due to falling levels of 25-OH vitamin D. It is reasonable to define vitamin D deficiency in the elderly at serum 25-OH vitamin D levels below 10 ng/ml. Vitamin D insufficiency has been determined as being less than 32 ng/ml. It is estimated that the daily amount of oral vitamin D needed to achieve adequate 25-OH vitamin D serum levels is approximately 2000 IU, with some estimating that double this amount would be required to ensure that the majority of the population maintained 25-OH vitamin D levels within the normal range.

The Health Effects of Low Vitamin D in the Elderly

Falls and Fractures

Falls in the elderly are multifactorial, resulting from neurological and musculoskeletal disorders, visual impairment, the effects of drugs and polypharmacy, as well as many environmental and external factors. Muscle weakness has been shown to be an important risk factor for falls. Vitamin D has important physiological effects on muscle function, acting on membrane receptors on the myocyte and on calcium uptake. Vitamin D deficiency may result in weakness of the proximal muscles causing a feeling of heaviness in the legs, tiring easily, and difficulty in walking up stairs and standing up from a sitting position.

Numerous studies have found a correlation between low serum 25-OH vitamin D in the elderly and muscle strength. Significant findings were a decrease in the power of leg extension, handgrip strength, inability to climb stairs, and falls. An associated reduction in walking distance has also been described. Nevertheless, in a healthy community dwelling older population, other studies found no significant differences in knee-extension strength in those lacking vitamin D.

A number of studies have attempted to show a correlation between vitamin D supplementation in patients with deficiency and the effect on muscle strength. The results of these studies have been equivocal. One study found that both knee extension strength and walking distance improved in women treated for 6 months by vitamin D supplementation [2]. Another study found that the functional ability of frail elderly subjects receiving vitamin D supplementation improved, and that they were able to dress in a shorter time [3]. However, in an inpatient population in a geriatric ward, supplementation did not improve activities of daily living.

Falls are common in advancing age, with approximately a third of older people falling at least once per year, and some 6-7% of these resulting in a fracture. Vitamin D deficiency has been reported to affect predominantly the weight-bearing antigravity muscles of the lower limbs, which are particularly important for walking and postural balance. Thus, it is not surprising that a correlation has been found between low serum 25-OH vitamin D levels and falls in the elderly. One study found that providing supplementation with vitamin D and calcium for as little as 8 weeks in those with vitamin D deficiency resulted in a decrease in body sway and falls over one year. However, a study in subjects 70 years and older receiving supplementation with 400 IU vitamin D_3 over 2 years failed to show significant benefits on reducing falls. Similarly, another study of a healthy elderly population receiving vitamin D and calcium over 3 years did not lower the incidence of falls compared to placebo.

An evaluation of the differences in the results of these studies raises a number of issues. It is clear that vitamin D has an important physiological role on muscular function, and thus has a direct effect on muscle strength, posture and balance. The correlation with vitamin D deficiency and decreased muscle strength and falls is probably more relevant in the frail elderly, where maintaining muscle strength and balance is more critical in preventing falls. In addition, the amount of vitamin D provided as supplementation in many of these studies was insufficient and unlikely to allow serum 25-OH vitamin D to reach adequate levels. It is thus important to evaluate the vitamin D status particularly in the frail elderly, and to provide them with adequate doses of vitamin D supplementation.

The subject of fracture prevention as a result of treatment with vitamin D and calcium supplementation has been well studied. While studies have shown increased bone density as a result of this therapy, the benefits in preventing osteoporotic fractures are controversial. In a large study of postmenopausal women in the Women's Health Initiative (WHI) clinical trial subjects were randomly assigned to receive a daily dose of either 1000 mg calcium with 400 IU vitamin D_3 or placebo. While hip bone density over an average follow-up period of 7 years improved significantly, hip fracture did not decrease significantly overall and there was an increased risk of kidney stones [4]. However, in those subjects with higher adherence to therapy, there was a significantly positive effect on reducing hip fractures. A meta-analysis published prior to this study found that oral vitamin D supplementation at doses 700 to 800IU/day appears to reduce the risk of hip and non-vertebral fractures in ambulatory or institutionalized older persons. The vitamin D dose is important, since a dose of 400 IU/day was found to be inadequate for the prevention of fractures [5]. Thus it seems that the possible benefit of vitamin D on osteoporotic fractures depends on the provision of an adequate dose on a regular basis.

Immune System

The vitamin D receptor (VDR) is a nuclear hormone receptor encoded by the VDR gene. This receptor is widely present on many tissues, such as muscle, neurons and glial cells, breast, colon, prostate, pancreatic β cells and immune cells. This explains the diverse effects of vitamin D on body functions. VDR is found on activated T cells, and vitamin D has an effect on immune function. Thus, not surprisingly, vitamin D has been shown to have a positive role in the immune response to tuberculosis. An association has been described with low levels of vitamin D and acute phase reactants and cytokine levels. In a study of older patients with heart failure lower levels of vitamin D were associated with raised levels of C-reactive protein (CRP). This was related to poorer physical performance and frailty. It remains unclear whether supplementation with vitamin D will have a positive effect on inflammatory markers.

Colon Cancer

The possible association between vitamin D and cancer is of great interest. The finding that the death rate from colon cancer in the USA was lowest in states of higher solar radiation, subsequently supported by population studies of disease incidence, raised the possibility of vitamin D being related to the development of colorectal cancer. The Nurses' Health Study found a 67% lower risk of colorectal cancer in women in the highest quintile of vitamin D intake. A number of studies have found that higher levels of serum 25-OH vitamin D are associated with a lower risk of colorectal cancer, particularly of the distal colon and rectum.

Breast Cancer

Epidemiological studies found lower rates of breast cancer mortality in sunny areas of the southern and southwestern USA, with the inverse association being strongest in urban areas. The Nurses' Health Study, however, did not find this geographic relationship for breast cancer incidence, adjusted for age and established risk factors. A subsequent case-control study based on death certificates did find a significantly reduced risk of breast cancer for those with higher sunlight exposure. The NHANES I study also found that increased sunlight exposure was associated with moderate reductions in breast cancer risk. There are limited data regarding serum levels of vitamin D and a possible reduced risk of breast cancer.

Prostate Cancer

Epidemiological studies suggest that higher levels of ambient UVB are associated with lower mortality rates from prostate cancer. In a case-control study of patients with prostate cancer and others with benign prostatic hypertrophy the risk of prostate cancer in those with cumulative lifetime sun exposure was significantly reduced. Another study found that sun exposure as well as VDR polymorphisms play important roles in the etiology of prostate cancer. Studies are inconclusive regarding the possible association between serum 25-OH vitamin D levels and cancer of the prostate. In fact, one study found a possible U-shaped association, with an increased risk of prostate cancer in men with the highest levels of 25-OH vitamin D. This raises the need for caution in providing high-dose supplementation over longer periods of time.

Ovarian Cancer and Non-Hodgkin's Lymphoma

Mortality from ovarian cancer has similarly been found to be negatively correlated with exposure to sunlight. Sunbathing and UV exposure is also associated with a decreased risk of non-Hodgkin's lymphoma. A high level of vitamin D at the time of diagnosis may improve the prognosis in this condition.

Cognitive Function

As mentioned earlier, vitamin D receptors (VDR) are present on neurons and glial cells. Thus vitamin D plays an important role in regulating functions such as neurotransmission, neuroprotection, neuro-immunomodulation and brain processes. VDR are found on cells in the cortex and hippocampus, which are important areas for cognitive function. Previous studies have suggested a positive role for vitamin D on cognitive function. In a systematic review evaluating the relationship between vitamin D and cognitive performance in adults, only five observational studies were included in the analysis [6]. No prospective cohort studies or randomized controlled studies were found. The results of the studies were inconclusive. While some found a significant positive association between serum 25-OH vitamin D concentrations and cognitive performance, in others no significant associations were found. This raises the need for more uniform methodology, cognitive assessments and randomized controlled trials to further evaluate this possible relationship.

Cardiovascular Disease and Mortality

There is accumulating evidence that low levels of vitamin D may have a detrimental effect on mortality. This has been found in those with end-stage renal disease and coronary artery disease. Since older adults are at higher risk for vitamin D deficiency, a prospective cohort study of those 65 years and older evaluated mortality in this population group. Baseline 25-OH vitamin D levels were inversely associated with cardiovascular and all-cause mortality.

Vitamin D Supplementation in the Elderly

The suggested dose of vitamin D for the older patient depends on baseline 25-OH vitamin D levels and on the clinical presentation. Standard doses of cholecalciferol of 400 – 600 IU daily are ineffective in raising 25-OH vitamin D levels. Daily doses of 2000 IU will increase levels to above 30ng/ml in approximately 85% of the population [7], whereas 5000 IU will achieve these levels in about 92% of the population [8]. While vitamin D is safe and toxicity is unlikely, the recommended daily dose for vitamin D supplementation in the elderly remains to be determined. A daily amount of 2000 IU to 3000 IU seems reasonable, and response can be monitored by serum levels.

Conclusion

Low levels of vitamin D are prevalent among older adults. There is great interest in the possible negative effects of this finding on the health and functional and cognitive abilities of the elderly. However, there is a need for more prospective studies designed to determine the benefits and doses of vitamin D supplementation in these conditions.

References

[1] Dawson-Hughes B, Heaney RP, Holick MF, Lips P, Meunier PJ, Vieth R. Estimates of optimal vitamin D status. *Osteoporos. Int.* 2005;16(7):713-6.

[2] Verhaar HJ, Samson MM, Jansen PA, de Vreede PL, Manten JW, Duursma SA. Muscle strength, functional mobility and vitamin D in older women. *Aging* (Milano). 2000;12(6):455-60.

[3] Gloth FM, 3rd, Smith CE, Hollis BW, Tobin JD. Functional improvement with vitamin D replenishment in a cohort of frail, vitamin D-deficient older people. *J. Am. Geriatr. Soc.* 1995;43(11):1269-71.

[4] Jackson RD, LaCroix AZ, Gass M, Wallace RB, Robbins J, Lewis CE, et al. Calcium plus vitamin D supplementation and the risk of fractures. *N. Engl. J. Med.* 2006;354(7):669-83.

[5] Bischoff-Ferrari HA, Willett WC, Wong JB, Giovannucci E, Dietrich T, Dawson-Hughes B. Fracture prevention with vitamin D supplementation: a meta-analysis of randomized controlled trials. *Jama.* 2005;293(18):2257-64.

[6] Annweiler C, Allali G, Allain P, Bridenbaugh S, Schott AM, Kressig RW, et al. Vitamin D and cognitive performance in adults: a systematic review. *Eur. J. Neurol.* 2009;16(10):1083-9.

[7] Heaney RP. Serum 25-hydroxyvitamin D and parathyroid hormone exhibit threshold behavior. *J. Endocrinol. Invest.* 2005;28(2):180-2.

[8] Mocanu V, Stitt PA, Costan AR, Voroniuc O, Zbranca E, Luca V, et al. Long-term effects of giving nursing home residents bread fortified with 125 microg (5000 IU) vitamin D(3) per daily serving. *Am. J. Clin. Nutr.* 2009;89(4):1132-7.

In: Vitamin D Deficiency
Editors: V. Lerner and C. Miodownik
ISBN: 978-1-61470-964-0

Chapter IX

Schizophrenia, Vitamin D and Autoimmunity — Are Low Serum Vitamin D Levels Related to Immune System Abnormalities? New Aspects and Review of the Literature

Dganit Itzhaky[1], Daniela Amital[2,3], Katya Gorden[3], Arnson Yoav[4], Alisa Bogomolni[1] and Howard Amital[2,4]

[1]Biochemistry and Immunology Labs, Meir Medical Center, Kfar Saba, Israel
[2]Sackler Faculty of Medicine, Tel Aviv University, Tel Aviv, Israel
[3]Department of Psychiatry 'B',
Ness Ziona Mental Health Center, Ness Ziona, Israel
[4] Department of Medicine 'B', Sheba Medical Center,
Tel-Hashomer, Israel. Affiliated with the Sackler Faculty of Medicine,
Tel Aviv University, Tel Aviv, Israel

Abstract

Aims: Vitamin D is increasingly associated with the pathology of cognition and mental illness. Vitamin D receptors have been detected on neurons that regulate behaviour. The aim of this study was to assess vitamin D serum concentrations in patients with major depression and schizophrenia compared to healthy controls and to determine if a correlation exists between serum levels of vitamin D and disease activity.

Methods: We recruited 50 patients with schizophrenia and as comparators we enrolled 33 patients with major depression and 50 controls with no major psychopathology. The Positive and Negative Syndrome Scale (PANSS) for schizophrenia and the Hamilton Depression scale for depression were administered at the same day the blood samples were drawn. We used LIAISON® 25 OH Vitamin D (DiaSorin) Immunoassay, to measure serum concentrations of 25 OH Vitamin D.

Results: Lower serum vitamin D concentrations were detected among patients with schizophrenia (15.0±7.3 ng/ml) compared to patients with depression (19.6±8.3ng/ml) and to controls (20.2±7.8 ng/ml, $p < 0.05$).We found no correlation between disease activity, measured by the PANSS score and vitamin D levels.

Conclusions: Lower serum vitamin D levels were found in patients with schizophrenia compared to patients with depression and to healthy controls. No correlation was found between serum concentration and disease activity. Additional studies are needed to elucidate the role of vitamin D in the autoimmune mechanism and in the pathogenesis of schizophrenia.

Keywords: Vitamin D, autoimmune diseases, schizophrenia, depression

Introduction

Schizophrenia is a mental disorder that affects up to 1% of the world population. The disease is characterized by progressive disintegration of cognitive and affective responsiveness leading to a major degree of personal, social, and vocational disability. The manifestations of the disease can be classified into positive symptoms (thought disorders, hallucinations, paranoia, and delusions), negative symptoms (social withdrawal, anhedonia, apathy, and paucity of speech), and cognitive impairments (deficits in perception, learning, attention, short and long-term memory, and executive function). Cognitive deficits are the primary disabilities associated with the illness and are a reliable predictor of long-term disability and treatment outcomes [1]. Even though the disease is so widely encountered, its etiology remains obscure.

Pathogenesis of Schizophrenia, the Immune Theory

Many mechanisms have been implicated in the pathogenesis of schizophrenia including neurodegenerative, neurotransmitter system abnormalities, central nervous system inflammation, altered genetic expression, obstetric complications, environmental influences, and immunological abnormalities including autoimmunity.

Schizophrenic patients suffer from alternating episodes of psychosis and remission, which lead to a steady continuous decline in social and cognitive functions. Many theories have been suggested to explain the remitting relapsing nature of the disease. Both the innate and adaptive arms of the immune system have been implicated to be involved in the immune dysfunction of schizophrenia (Table 1) [2].

Anti-neuronal antibodies have been reported in "classical" autoimmune disorders such as systemic lupus erythematosus and Sjogren's syndrome, particularly when coexisting neurological and psychiatric manifestations appear [3-6]. These antibodies are often associated with cognitive deficits and psychosis. In particular, anti-cerebral muscarinic cholinergic receptors associated with central nervous system (CNS) alterations have been described in Sjogren's syndrome [7].

Table 1. Immune system abnormalities associated with schizophrenia

Non specific Autoantibodies elevated in association with Schizophrenia	Anticardiolipin, Antinuclear, anti-DNA, anti-Histone
Specific Autoantibodies against brain structures	Ab against the hippocampus, septum, cingulated gyrus, amygdala and frontal cortex
Th1/Th2 imbalance	T-helper type 1 activation, Increased IL-2, Increased IL-2 receptors, Elevated IL-6. T-Helper type 2 activation, Increased IL-4 and IL-10 (in several studies).
Infections	Increased serum and CSF Ab against HSV, CMV, EBV, measles, retrovirus, Bornavirus.
Association with other autoimmune conditions	High rates of Graves' disease, intestinal malabsorption, acquired hemolytic anemia, interstitial cystitis, and Sjogren's syndrome

Autoimmune mechanisms have been implicated in the pathogenesis of schizophrenia [8-11]. Several studies have elaborated on the various immunological aspects detected among schizophrenic patients, including antibodies to neurotransmitter receptors and cytokines [12-14], and the appearance of antinuclear antibodies (ANA) in patients with schizophrenia along with increased concentrations of IL-3 producing CD5+ B cells [15-19]. Other autoimmune aspects of schizophrenia are believed to occur following viral infections. Second-trimester exposure to poliovirus infection and childhood exposure to common infections have been suggested as risk factors for future development of schizophrenia [20-22]. The most studied indirect evidence of autoimmune etiology of schizophrenia is from the neuropsychiatric involvement in SLE.

Many observations link autoimmunity to infections. One proposed mechanisms is based on molecular mimicry, a structural homology between the pathogenic agent and a host protein that provokes an auto-reactive response [23-27]. The blood-brain barrier (BBB) may have a critical role in the development of schizophrenia because it normally separates the CNS from invading pathogens as well as from deleterious components of the immune response [28]. Individual differences in BBB development are presumably determined by genetic, as well as by maternal factors such as intrauterine hypoxia [29]. The BBB is a complex structure comprised of multiple cell types, and its ability to exclude infectious agents and harmful immune influences is poorly understood [30]. A delay in a crucial aspect of BBB development could leave the immature brain vulnerable to pathogens that have the capacity to provoke a cascade of host responses, such as the secretion of pro-inflammatory cytokines. These molecules might disrupt normal neurodevelopment in fetal brains unshielded by the BBB, thus leading to pre-schizophrenic neuro-circuitry alterations. Interestingly, substantial portions (7%–33%) of schizophrenic patients have evidence of BBB abnormalities [31] that do not appear to be related to antipsychotic medications [32]. Nonetheless, according to certain neurodevelopmental theories, a defect in the BBB would be expected to precede schizophrenia. Although many possible pathophysiological mechanisms might result in BBB impairment, only a minority of patients with schizophrenia actively manifest BBB abnormalities after the disorder is diagnosed.

Five autoimmune disorders appear more frequently in schizophrenia patients prior to the onset of the illness: Graves' disease, intestinal malabsorption, acquired hemolytic anemia, interstitial cystitis, and Sjogren's syndrome [33]. Immune system abnormalities such as atypical lymphocytes, similar to those found in infectious mononucleosis and other viral diseases, autoantibodies, and increased levels of pro-inflammatory cytokines were reported in patients with schizophrenia. These immune alterations could lead to inflammatory insult in the brain. Indeed, some studies have demonstrated microglial activation, inflammatory signs, and upregulation of inflammatory genes in the brains of patients with schizophrenia. Elevated serum PGE_2 induces enhanced production of IL-6, which is consistently increased in schizophrenia [34].

Increased antibody titers have been detected in schizophrenic patients. One explanation is that these patients are predisposed to more vigorous B-cell responses and consequently prone to develop autoantibodies. Studies of lymphocyte subsets in schizophrenia patients found an increase in B cells, and a subset of patients with elevated number of CD5+ B cells, which are thought to be involved in autoantibody production. Nevertheless, these data have not been consistently replicated.

Evidence of impaired immune responses in schizophrenic patients has also been reported [31]. Controversy also surrounds data from various laboratories that have demonstrated autoantibodies against brain components of schizophrenic patients. Several brain regions may be targets of autoimmune reactions. In a recent study, anti-hippocampal antibodies were found to correlate with low IL-2 responses, suggesting an autoimmune phenotype in a subgroup of schizophrenia patients [35].

The muscarinic cholinergic (mACh) system is one of the most crucial neuro-immunomodulators in the CNS. Cholinergic neurons have projections that make synaptic contact with highly specific targets in a variety of regions including the cortex. Factors that are able to modify cholinergic transmission have been implicated in the manifestation of schizophrenia [36]. Antibodies against muscarinic acetylcholine receptors (mAChR) have been shown to induce cholinergic nitric oxide synthase (NOS) activation and generation of prostaglandin-E2 (PGE2) and metalloproteioase-3(MMP-3). It is possible that the immune response exerted by these autoantibodies might lead to deregulation of cerebral mAChR functional activity and cerebral inflammation. Autoantibodies that display agonistic activity may trigger NO, PGE_2, and MMP-3 production.

Inflammatory processes in the brain lead to the induction of MMP-3, which is highly destructive and attacks several extracellular matrix molecules [37]. MMP-3 is localized in macrophage-like cells and is found mainly in neurons and microglia. The proinflammatory action of anti-M1 mAChR autoantibodies and the role of serum autoantibodies against mAChR as a neuro-immune factor are considered in the etiology of schizophrenia, possibly explaining the presence of circulating antibodies from patients with paranoid schizophrenia. The antibodies can inhibit irreversible binding of the specific mAChR radio-ligand. M5 or M2 mAChR activation by autoantibodies can give conflicting messages. Chronic autoantibody fixation on postsynaptic neuronal M1 mAChR results in receptor downregulation, uncoupled to Gq protein, which stabilizes phospholipase C activity, interferes with cognitive function (including attention, learning and memory), and alters neuronal plasticity, which causes negative symptoms. On the other hand, the antibody binding to presynaptic glia M2 mAChR inhibits the activation of these receptors ending up with reduced excitatory neurotransmitter release (dopamine and glutamate). Therefore, the antibodies could induce loss of glial physiological buffering functions, which might cause additional positive symptoms.

The autoimmune hypothesis for schizophrenia is not limited to autoantibody formation or cytokines crossing the BBB. Some studies have shown other immunological alterations in schizophrenia [43], demonstrating the potential importance of host responses to pathogens in determining disease expression. Viruses and other infections can promote or trigger autoimmune diseases of the nervous system, sometimes after a long latency period. There are assumptions that immunogenetic factors play a role in determining which infected individuals succumb to virus-elicited autoimmune diseases. For example, only a small portion of people infected with HTLV-I develop tropical spastic paraparesis (HTLV-I associated myelopathy) but the risk of this latent complication is correlated with specific host HLA haplotypes [38]. Associations between HLA types and schizophrenia (or subtypes of the disease) have also been reported [31] and these findings could be relevant to viral infections *in utero* because expression of major histocompatability genes is evident by the beginning of the second trimester [39]. Thus, schizophrenia could be initiated by an endemic virus that causes neuropsychiatric sequelae only in individuals who are genetically predisposed to mount an atypical immune response during a critical neurodevelopmental period. In this regard, cytokines and growth factors could be critical intermediates in this process at various stages of disease development [40].

The mechanism of action of antipsychotic drugs suggests that schizophrenic manifestations are based on over-stimulation or blockade of normal neurotransmissions [41]. The antipsychotic effect involves blocking dopamine D2 activity and affinity of the drug for mAChR. Therefore, schizophrenia is not likely to be explained by an excess or deficiency of a single neurotransmitter, but rather by abnormalities in several transmitter systems and in particular the delicate interaction between dopaminergic and cholinergic systems in various regions of the brain. These interactions are particularly significant in regions considered relevant in schizophrenia, such as the frontal cortex. There is also considerable evidence of extensive interactions between the dopaminergic and cholinergic systems. The M1 mAChR in particular may be involved in modulation of excitatory amino acid neurotransmissions in cortical and limbic areas [42]. Therefore, the cholinergic system is relevant to the cause of schizophrenia and has a role in the symptomatic treatment of the disease.

Vitamin D Levels and Abnormalities of the Central Nervous System

Several authors have investigated the link between vitamin D and the CNS. Vitamin D is increasingly associated with cognitive abilities; lower levels of vitamin D were significantly more prevalent among patients with multiple sclerosis and preceded the development of the disease by years [43;44]. Vitamin D receptors have been detected on neurons that take part in behavior control and regulation. Vitamin D supplementation during early fetal growth and early childhood had a positive effect on brain development and on later mental functioning [45-47].

Vitamin D regulates the immune system in several mechanisms (Table 2), and low vitamin D levels were found to be a risk factor for several diseases, including conditions involving the central nervous system. A study investigating bone metabolism in multiple sclerosis (MS) patients revealed a prevalence of insufficient serum 25(OH)D levels (<50 nmol/l) in 77% of patients [48]. Munger et al. [49] reported that among white, active-duty, US military personnel, the risk of developing multiple sclerosis (MS) significantly decreased with increasing levels of 25-hydroxyvitamin D. Another study checked the vitamin D intake in more than 187,000 women from two separate cohorts, the Nurses' Health Study (NHS; 92,253 women followed from 1980 to 2000) and Nurses' Health Study II (NHS II; 95,310 women followed from 1991 to 2001). They found a 40% reduction in risk of MS among women who took supplemental vitamin D, primarily in the form of multivitamins, compared with women who did not take supplements [50].

Table 2. Immune-regulatory effects of vitamin D

Effects on Th1/Th2 balance	Inhibition of T lymphocyte proliferation, particularly of the Th1 arm. Inhibition of cytokine production. Decreased secretion of IL-2 and IFN-γ , enhanced IL-5 and IL-10 production.
Effects on B-cells	Inhibition of antibody secretion and autoantibody production.
Effects antigen presenting cells	Inhibits the differentiation of monocytes into dendritic cells and impedes the stimulatory activity that T cells exert on them.
Effects on Macrophages	Decrease of the antigen presenting activity to lymphocytes. Increased expression of macrophage specific surface antigens and the lysosomal enzyme acid phosphatase.

A recent study conducted among 3,173 individuals aged 50 to 79 years and free of Parkinson disease demonstrated that subjects with higher serum vitamin D concentrations showed a reduced risk for Parkinson disease. The relative risk between the highest and lowest quartiles was 0.33 (95% confidence interval (CI), 0.14-0.80) after adjustment for sex, age, marital status, education, alcohol consumption, leisure-time physical activity, smoking, body mass index, and month of blood draw [51].

Few studies have examined the putative association between serum vitamin D concentration and mental illness. Two reports explored the linkage between vitamin D and osteoporosis in patients with schizophrenia [52;53]. While two teams recorded low vitamin D concentrations among this population [54;55], another study detected values that equaled those in the control group [56]. A study conducted in Denmark demonstrated that neonates with low vitamin D concentrations had a significantly increased risk of schizophrenia (up to 2-fold) compared to neonates with concentrations ranging between 40.5 and 50.9 nmol/L. Interestingly, neonates with excessive concentrations of vitamin D also had an elevated risk for this disorder [57]. Additional epidemiological data underlines an increased prevalence of schizophrenia among winter newborns [58], which may be attributable to low vitamin D levels occurring more often during that season.

Data regarding vitamin D levels among the Israeli population of psychiatric patients are lacking. Therefore, the aim of this study was to assess vitamin D levels in patients with major depression and schizophrenia compared to healthy controls. Possible correlations between serum concentrations of vitamin D and disease activity were also investigated. As a comparator, standard autoimmune parameters such as anti-cardiolipin antibodies (IgG, IgM) were measured to determine their possible involvement in the emergence of schizophrenia.

Material and Methods

Patient Sera

Sera were collected at the Ness Ziona Mental Health Center, Israel. Study subjects included 50 patients with schizophrenia, 33 patients with major depression, and 50 controls (health centre staff) with no major psychopathology. All subjects were age-matched adults who consented to take part in the study, which was approved by the local ethical committee.

Clinical and psychiatric evaluations

1) Demographic details including age, gender, BMI, ethnicity, occupation, living arrangements, and marital status were recorded.
2) Subjective estimation of daily duration of sun exposure.
3) Clinical manifestations of disease, including diagnosis, age at first psychiatric diagnosis, number of hospitalizations, duration and type of psychiatric and other medications used, and family mental health history.

Medications: To rule out a possible effect of medications as causing the difference in vitamin D levels between the three groups, patients were categorized according to medications used. The schizophrenic patients were divided into 4 different subgroups according to different combinations of medications, antipsychotic, mood stabilizers, etc. A single patient out of 50 was not taking any medication.

1) Nutritional assessment (fish and oils, meat, eggs). Each patient completed a dietary assessment regarding his or her intake of vitamin D containing foods.
2) Clinical assessment. The Clinical Global Impression (CGI) Scale was used to evaluate the participants' level of general functioning. The CGI is a standardized assessment tool that allows the clinician to rate illness severity. The scale consists of three global subscales formatted for use with the Global Scoring Sheet. Values are scored on a Likert scale ranging from 1 to 7.

Mental Health Assessment. The Positive and Negative Syndrome Scale (PANSS) for schizophrenia and the Hamilton Depression Scale were administered the same day the blood sample was drawn. These are validated scales and customarily used to quantify the intensity of psychotic and depressive conditions, respectively.

Briefly, the PANSS is used for measuring symptom severity of patients with schizophrenia and for evaluation of positive and negative symptoms of psychotic disorders [59].

The Hamilton Depression Scale is used to rate the severity of depression in patients who have been diagnosed as depressed. The higher the score, the more severe the depression [60].

Vitamin D measurement. The LIAISON® 25 OH Vitamin D (DiaSorin) Immunoassay was used to measure serum concentration of 25 OH Vitamin D. This method for quantitative determination of 25-OH vitamin D is a direct, competitive, chemiluminescent immunoassay. A specific antibody to vitamin D is used to coat magnetic particles (solid phase) and vitamin D is linked to an isoluminol derivative. During incubation, 25-OH vitamin D is dissociated from its binding protein and competes with labeled vitamin D for binding sites on the antibody. After incubation, the unbound material is removed with a wash cycle. Subsequently, the starter reagents are added and a flash chemiluminescent reaction is initiated. The light signal is measured by a photomultiplier as relative light units (RLU) and is inversely proportional to the concentration of 25-OH vitamin D present in calibrators, controls, or samples.

Anti-Cardiolipin IgM and IgG antibody measurement was conducted using the LIAISON® for quantitative determination of the autoantibody titers. This is a two-step immuno-luminometric sandwich assay using directly coated magnetic microparticles.

Statistical Analysis. Prevalence rates between the groups were compared using chi-square and Fisher exact tests (two-tailed), as appropriate. Continuous variables are expressed as mean ± standard deviation (SD), and were compared between the three groups by one-way ANOVA with multiple comparisons by Bonferroni. Student's t-test was used to compare continuous variables in two groups. Pearson correlations were performed for associations between variables. We used multiple linear regression tests to look for predictive variables for anti-cardiolipin antibody levels. For all tests, a *p*–value <0.05 was considered statistically significant. SPSS–17 was used for data analysis.

Results

Patients

Patients with Schizophrenia. Overall, 50 patients with schizophrenia were enrolled. Their average age was 40.2±13.4 years (range 19-65 years). There were 34 males (68%) and 16 (32%) females. The mean age of disease onset was 24.8±10.5 years and disease duration was an average of 15.4±12.6 years. The average overall PANSS score was 22.5 ± 8.5; the positive psychotic symptoms score was 19.6 ± 8.1 and the negative symptoms score was 28.6 ± 7.7.

Patients with Major Depression. As a comparator, 33 patients with major depression were enrolled. One patient was eliminated from the study because of technical problems with the laboratory testing. The average age was 48.5±11.4 years (range 18-65 years), with 11 males (33%) and 22 (67%) females. The mean age at disease onset was 48.4±11.8 years and disease duration was 10.2±10.4 years. The average Hamilton score was 19.1±11.0.

Healthy controls. As a second comparator, 50 healthy controls, 13 males (26%) and 37 (74%) females, at an average age of 39.7±10.7 years were recruited.

As expected, the healthy controls assessed their CGI at X.0, whereas patients with schizophrenia had more severe disease, reflected by a CGI score of 5.6±0.9, compared to patients with depression 3.6±1.4, (p<0.01).

Daily duration of sun exposure There were no significant differences in the average patient estimates of daily sun exposure; patients with schizophrenia estimated time spent exposed to sun as 1.7±2.2 hours, compared to patients with depression(1.0±1.0 hours), and healthy controls (1.2±1.2 hours; Table 3).

Effect of Nutrition on Vitamin D Concentrations

There was no significant difference in diet composition regarding vitamin D containing elements. There was a minor difference in egg consumption (92% of schizophrenic patients compared to 76% of depression patients) but the correlation to vitamin D serum concentration was borderline ($p=0.08$).

Table 3. Average daily sun exposure (in hours) estimated by study subjects

Group	No. of subjects	Sun exposure (hours) Mean±SD	P value
Healthy Controls	50	1.2±1.2	Not significant
Depression	32	1.0±1.0	
Schizophrenia	50	1.7±2.2	

Within the schizophrenic group, we found higher vitamin D concentrations between those who ate fish 17.3±8.2 ng/ml (25 patients) compared to those who did not 11.7±5.4 ng/ml (24 patients) ($p=0.02$).

According to the nutrition survey, four patients in the depression group and one of the healthy controls consumed vitamin D supplements.

Vitamin D Serum Concentrations

Patients with schizophrenia had significantly lower serum vitamin D levels compared to patients with depression and to controls (15.0±7.3, 19.6±8.3 and 20.2±7.8 ng/ml, respectively; $p<0.05$). There was no significant difference between vitamin D levels in the depression group compared to healthy controls (Figure 1).

Table 4. Vitamin D status according to levels in the study population ($P<0.05$)

Vitamin D status	Group N (%)			
	Schizophrenia	Depression	Controls	Total
Deficient (<15 ng/ml)	28 (57.1)	11 (33.3)	12 (24.5)	51 (39.0)
Insufficient (15-30 ng/ml)	20 (40.8)	18 (54.5)	31 (63.3)	69 (53.0)
Sufficient (> 30ng/ml)	1 (2.0)	4 (12.0)	6 (12.2)	11 (8.0)

N=number of subjects. %= percentage of subjects.

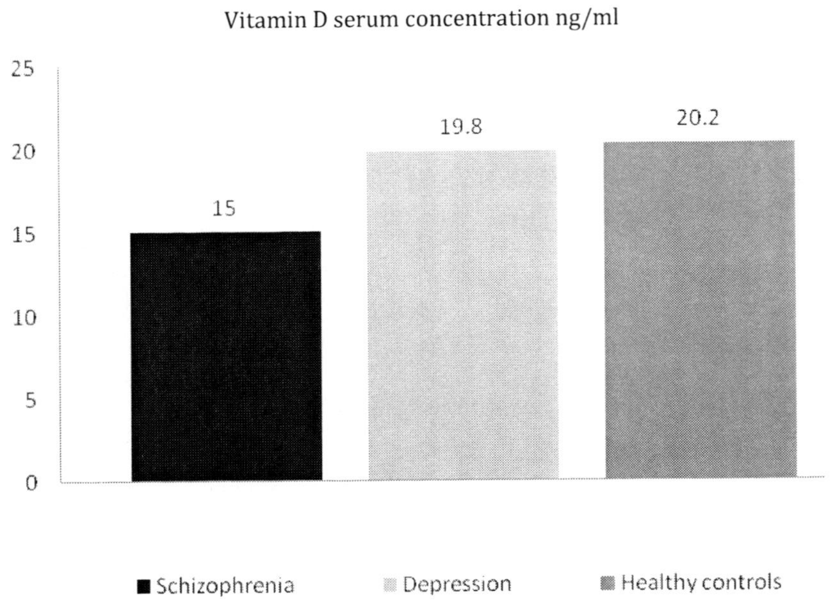

Figure 1. Concentration of vitamin D according to study group.

When patients were grouped according to vitamin D levels (deficient: below 15 ng/ml, insufficient: 15-30ng/ml, or sufficient: above 30 ng/ml) the schizophrenia group comprised a greater proportion 28/49 (57.1%) of all vitamin D deficient patients compared to vitamin D insufficient patients 20/49 (40.8%; Table 3).

Vitamin D Levels and Concomitant Medications

To analyze the possible effects of concomitant medications on serum vitamin D concentrations, drugs were classified into four main categories: antipsychotics, antidepressants, sedatives, and mood stabilizers. There was no relationship between medication types or combinations with vitamin D serum concentration (data not shown).

Vitamin D levels and disease activity. The level of vitamin D did not correlate with disease duration, CGI scores, or PANSS scores.

Cardiovascular morbidity. Analysis of non-psychiatric clinical manifestations showed a greater proportion of cardiovascular disease present in the patient groups compared to controls. Because cardiovascular disease has been associated with low vitamin D levels, we investigated this in our population.

All subjects were categorized according to cardiovascular medical history. Significantly lower vitamin D concentrations were found among patients with depression and existing cardiovascular disease (Table 5).

Anti-cardiolipin antibody levels. There was no difference between the three study groups regarding anti-cardiolipin IgG (IgGaCl) or IgM (IgMaCl) levels.

Table 5. Association between concomitant cardiovascular disease and vitamin D serum concentrations

Group	Cardiovascular disease	No. of subjects*	Vitamin D ng/ml	P value
Controls	no	45	19.9±7.8	0.434
	yes	4	23.1±7.8	
Depression	no	20	21.6±8.9	0.043
	yes	8	14.4±4.9	
Schizophrenia	no	39	14.6±7.5	0.408
	yes	9	16.9±7.0	

IgGaCl levels in the schizophrenia group did not differ from those recorded in patients with depression or with the healthy controls, at 4.1±8.3, 2.6±1.8, and 3.5±5.2 U/ml, respectively. Similarly, IgMaCl levels in the three study groups were 3.8±7.6, 2.4±1.0, and 2.9±2.1 U/ml, respectively.

In the schizophrenia group, disease activity (PANSS) correlated with cardiolipin IgM antibody titers (p=0.012).

Discussion

The etiology of schizophrenia is multifactorial. Acquired, genetic and environmental factors, as well as infections and autoimmune reactivity have been implicated in its pathogenesis [22;61;62]. Vitamin D is believed to have therapeutic benefits; it has been reported that vitamin D activates receptors on neurons located in regions involved with behavior regulation, stimulates neurotrophin release, and protects the brain by enhancing antioxidant and anti-inflammatory defenses against vascular injury [63].

Our results indicate that adults with schizophrenia had significantly lower serum concentrations of vitamin D compared to healthy controls and to patients suffering from major depression. This finding remained after evaluating the impact of various factors such as self-reported sun exposure, consumption of various medications and food supplements, and analysis of diet composition.

One would expect that vitamin D levels in schizophrenic patients in Israel would be relatively high due to the sunny climate. However, patients in our study were recruited from a closed psychiatric ward, where mobility is restricted. It is likely that most of these patients estimated their daily sun exposure based on levels achieved prior to hospitalization, when they were recruited for this study. Patients with depression had vitamin D levels similar to those of the controls. This cohort was more heterogeneous than the patients with schizophrenia were; some patients were recruited from the outpatient clinic, reflecting less severe disease. Therefore, it seems reasonable that their daily habits and activities were similar to those of the healthy controls, leading to comparable vitamin D levels.

Vitamin D is involved in many metabolic functions in addition to bone and calcium metabolism; diverse cells carry vitamin D receptors on their membranes [64-72]. There is mounting evidence that vitamin D supplementation reduces overall mortality [73]. Other reports (mainly retrospective) indicate that adequate vitamin D serum levels are associated with protection from various malignancies, thromboses and cardiovascular diseases [74-76]. Vitamin D has also been observed to confer a moderating effect on the immune system by restraining overactive states of different immune cells [77;78]. Vitamin D deficiency was found to be related to autoimmunity and immune cell over-activity, and to be associated with animal models of diabetes, rheumatoid arthritis, and other autoimmune disorders [79-91].

Despite the low vitamin D concentrations we observed in patients with schizophrenia, we failed to demonstrate a correlation between vitamin D levels and disease activity measured by the PANSS score, which estimates the severity of the condition. This score is well-validated for schizophrenia [92], however it does not seem to touch on the relevant aspects that associate this condition with vitamin D concentration.

There was a high prevalence of cardiovascular diseases in the patient groups compared to controls (Figure 2). High risk for cardiovascular disease has been reported in depression and schizophrenia [93;94]. An inverse association between vitamin D concentrations and comorbid cardiovascular conditions was found in the depression subgroup only (Table 4). This may be related to their higher average age and higher rates of cardiovascular morbidity measured in this study.

Although some studies found that autoimmune mechanisms may be involved in the pathogenesis of schizophrenia [95], we did not find elevated titers of aCl antibodies level in our patient groups. Our findings are compatible with previous publications, yet the literature varies regarding this issue [96;97]. Our study detected a positive correlation (although within normal levels) of anticardiolipin antibody titers and severity of schizophrenia. The significance of this finding needs to be investigated further.

In conclusion, low serum vitamin D levels may play a role in the pathogenesis of schizophrenia. Based on our findings, we advocate routine testing of vitamin D levels in these patients and supplementation as needed. Additional studies are warranted to confirm the relationship between other implications of our study, such as anticardiolipin antibodies, and cardiovascular manifestations to the mechanisms of autoimmune involvement in schizophrenia.

References

[1] Meltzer,H.Y. (1999) Treatment of schizophrenia and spectrum disorders: pharmacotherapy, psychosocial treatments, and neurotransmitter interactions. *Biol. Psychiatry*, 46, 1321-1327.

[2] Jones,A.L., Mowry,B.J., Pender,M.P. and Greer,J.M. (2005) Immune dysregulation and self-reactivity in schizophrenia: do some cases of schizophrenia have an autoimmune basis? *Immunol. Cell Biol.*, 83, 9-17.

[3] Amital-Teplizki,H., Avinoach,I., Coates,A.R., Kooperman,O., Blank,M. and Shoenfeld,Y. (1989) Binding of monoclonal anti-DNA and anti-TB glycolipids to brain tissue. *Autoimmunity*, 4, 277-287.

[4] Avinoach,I., mital-Teplizki,H., Kuperman,O., Isenberg,D.A. and Shoenfeld,Y. (1990) Characteristics of antineuronal antibodies in systemic lupus erythematosus patients with

and without central nervous system involvement: the role of mycobacterial cross-reacting antigens. *Isr. J. Med. Sci.*, 26, 367-373.

[5] Colburn,K.K., Green,L.M. and Wong,A.K. (2001) Circulating antibodies to guanosine in systemic lupus erythematosus: correlation with nephritis and polyserositis by acute and longitudinal analyses. *Lupus*, 10, 410-417.

[6] Orman,B., Sterin-Borda,L., De Couto,P.A., Reina,S. and Borda,E. (2007) Anti-brain cholinergic auto antibodies from primary Sjogren syndrome sera modify simultaneously cerebral nitric oxide and prostaglandin biosynthesis. *Int. Immunopharmacol.*, 7, 1535-1543.

[7] Orman,B., Sterin-Borda,L., De Couto,P.A., Reina,S. and Borda,E. (2007) Anti-brain cholinergic auto antibodies from primary Sjogren syndrome sera modify simultaneously cerebral nitric oxide and prostaglandin biosynthesis. *Int. Immunopharmacol.*, 7, 1535-1543.

[8] Goldsmith,C.A. and Rogers,D.P. (2008) The case for autoimmunity in the etiology of schizophrenia. *Pharmacotherapy*, 28, 730-741.

[9] Moscavitch,S.D., Szyper-Kravitz,M. and Shoenfeld,Y. (2009) Autoimmune pathology accounts for common manifestations in a wide range of neuro-psychiatric disorders: the olfactory and immune system interrelationship. *Clin. Immunol.*, 130, 235-243.

[10] Spivak,B., Radwan,M., Bartur,P., Mester,R. and Weizman,A. (1995) Antinuclear autoantibodies in chronic schizophrenia. *Acta Psychiatr. Scand.*, 92, 266-269.

[11] Strous,R.D. and Shoenfeld,Y. (2006) Schizophrenia, autoimmunity and immune system dysregulation: a comprehensive model updated and revisited. *J. Autoimmun.*, 27, 71-80.

[12] Matsunaga,H., Tanaka,S., Fukumori,A., Tomonaga,K., Ikuta,K., Amino,N. et al (2008) Isotype analysis of human anti-Borna disease virus antibodies in Japanese psychiatric and general population. *J. Clin. Virol.*, 43, 317-322.

[13] Strous,R.D. and Shoenfeld,Y. (2006) Schizophrenia, autoimmunity and immune system dysregulation: a comprehensive model updated and revisited. *J. Autoimmun.*, 27, 71-80.

[14] Tanaka,S., Matsunaga,H., Kimura,M., Tatsumi,K., Hidaka,Y., Takano,T., et al. (2003) Autoantibodies against four kinds of neurotransmitter receptors in psychiatric disorders. *J. Neuroimmunol.*, 141, 155-164.

[15] Ganguli,R., Rabin,B.S. and Brar,J.S. (1992) Antinuclear and gastric parietal cell autoantibodies in schizophrenic patients. *Biol. Psychiatry*, 32, 735-738.

[16] 16.Ganguli,R., Brar,J.S., Chengappa,K.N., Yang,Z.W., Nimgaonkar,V.L. and Rabin,B.S. (1993) Autoimmunity in schizophrenia: a review of recent findings. *Ann. Med*, 25, 489-496.

[17] Sirota,P., Schild,K., Elizur,A., Djaldetti,M. and Fishman,P. (1995) Increased interleukin-1 and interleukin-3 like activity in schizophrenic patients. *Prog. Neuropsychopharmacol. Biol. Psychiatry*, 19, 75-83.

[18] Spivak,B., Radwan,M., Elimelech,D., Baruch,Y., Avidan,G. and Tyano,S. (1989) A study of the complement system in psychiatric patients. *Biol. Psychiatry*, 26, 640-642.

[19] Spivak,B., Radwan,M., Bartur,P., Mester,R. and Weizman,A. (1995) Antinuclear autoantibodies in chronic schizophrenia. *Acta Psychiatr. Scand.*, 92, 266-269.

[20] Brown,A.S. (2010) The environment and susceptibility to schizophrenia. *Prog. Neurobiol.*.

[21] Suvisaari,J., Haukka,J., Tanskanen,A., Hovi,T. and Lonnqvist,J. (1999) Association between prenatal exposure to poliovirus infection and adult schizophrenia. *Am. J. Psychiatry*, 156, 1100-1102.

[22] Suvisaari,J. (2010) [Risk factors of schizophrenia]. *Duodecim*, 126, 869-876.

[23] Amital,H., Govoni,M., Maya,R., Meroni,P.L., Ori,B., Shoenfeld,Y., et al. (2008) Role of infectious agents in systemic rheumatic diseases. *Clin. Exp. Rheumatol.*, 26, S27-S32.

[24] Arnson,Y., Amital,H., Guiducci,S., Matucci-Cerinic,M., Valentini,G., Barzilai,O., Maya,R. et al. (2009) The role of infections in the immunopathogensis of systemic sclerosis--evidence from serological studies. *Ann. N. Y. Acad. Sci.*, 1173, 627-632.

[25] Grossman,C., Dovrish,Z., Shoenfeld,Y. and Amital,H. (2010) Do infections facilitate the emergence of systemic sclerosis? *Autoimmun. Rev.*

[26] Plot,L. and Amital,H. (2009) Infectious associations of Celiac disease. *Autoimmun. Rev.*, 8, 316-319.

[27] Plot,L., Amital,H., Barzilai,O., Ram,M., Nicola,B. and Shoenfeld,Y. (2009) Infections may have a protective role in the etiopathogenesis of celiac disease. *Ann. N. Y. Acad. Sci.*, 1173, 670-674.

[28] Fabry,Z., Raine,C.S. and Hart,M.N. (1994) Nervous tissue as an immune compartment: the dialect of the immune response in the CNS. *Immunol. Today*, 15, 218-224.

[29] Goldstein,G.W., Robertson,P. and Betz,A.L. (1988) Update on the role of the blood-brain barrier in damage to immature brain. *Pediatrics*, 81, 732-734.

[30] Fabry,Z., Raine,C.S. and Hart,M.N. (1994) Nervous tissue as an immune compartment: the dialect of the immune response in the CNS. *Immunol. Today*, 15, 218-224.

[31] Kirch,D.G. (1993) Infection and autoimmunity as etiologic factors in schizophrenia: a review and reappraisal. *Schizophr. Bull.*, 19, 355-370.

[32] Kirch,D.G., Alexander,R.C., Suddath,R.L., Papadopoulos,N.M., Kaufmann,C.A., Daniel,D.G. et al. (1992) Blood-CSF barrier permeability and central nervous system immunoglobulin G in schizophrenia. *J. Neural. Transm. Gen. Sect.*, 89, 219-232.

[33] Eaton,W.W., Byrne,M., Ewald,H., Mors,O., Chen,C.Y., Agerbo,E. a et al. (2006) Association of schizophrenia and autoimmune diseases: linkage of Danish national registers. *Am. J. Psychiatry*, 163, 521-528.

[34] Muller,N. and Schwarz,M.J. (2010) Immune System and Schizophrenia. *Curr. Immunol. Rev.*, 6, 213-220.

[35] Yang,Z.W., Chengappa,K.N., Shurin,G., Brar,J.S., Rabin,B.S., Gubbi,A.V. et al. (1994) An association between anti-hippocampal antibody concentration and lymphocyte production of IL-2 in patients with schizophrenia. *Psychol. Med*, 24, 449-455.

[36] Saetre,P., Emilsson,L., Axelsson,E., Kreuger,J., Lindholm,E. and Jazin,E. (2007) Inflammation-related genes up-regulated in schizophrenia brains. *BMC. Psychiatry*, 7, 46.

[37] Rosenberg,G.A. (2002) Matrix metalloproteinases in neuroinflammation. *Glia*, 39, 279-291.

[38] Jeffery,K.J., Usuku,K., Hall,S.E., Matsumoto,W., Taylor,G.P., Procter,J., et al. (1999) HLA alleles determine human T-lymphotropic virus-I (HTLV-I) proviral load and the risk of HTLV-I-associated myelopathy. *Proc. Natl. Acad. Sci. USA*, 96, 3848-3853.

[39] Hofman,F.M., Danilovs,J.A. and Taylor,C.R. (1984) HLA-DR (Ia)-positive dendritic-like cells in human fetal nonlymphoid tissues. *Transplantation*, 37, 590-594.

[40] Nawa,H., Takahashi,M. and Patterson,P.H. (2000) Cytokine and growth factor involvement in schizophrenia--support for the developmental model. *Mol. Psychiatry*, 5, 594-603.

[41] Jones,A.L., Mowry,B.J., Pender,M.P. and Greer,J.M. (2005) Immune dysregulation and self-reactivity in schizophrenia: do some cases of schizophrenia have an autoimmune basis? *Immunol. Cell Biol.*, 83, 9-17.

[42] Bymaster,F.P., Shannon,H.E., Rasmussen,K., DeLapp,N.W., Ward,J.S., Calligaro,D.O., et al (1999) Potential role of muscarinic receptors in schizophrenia. *Life Sci.*, 64, 527-534.

[43] Munger,K.L., Zhang,S.M., O'Reilly,E., Hernan,M.A., Olek,M.J., Willett,W.C. et al. (2004) Vitamin D intake and incidence of multiple sclerosis. *Neurology*, 62, 60-65.

[44] Munger,K.L., Levin,L.I., Hollis,B.W., Howard,N.S. and Ascherio,A. (2006) Serum 25-hydroxyvitamin D levels and risk of multiple sclerosis. *JAMA*, 296, 2832-2838.

[45] Eyles,D.W., Smith,S., Kinobe,R., Hewison,M. and McGrath,J.J. (2005) Distribution of the vitamin D receptor and 1 alpha-hydroxylase in human brain. *J Chem. Neuroanat.*, 29, 21-30.

[46] Eyles,D.W., Feron,F., Cui,X., Kesby,J.P., Harms,L.H., Ko,P., et al. (2009) Developmental vitamin D deficiency causes abnormal brain development. *Psychoneuroendocrinology*, 34 Suppl 1, S247-S257.

[47] McGrath,J.J., Feron,F.P., Burne,T.H., kay-Sim,A. and Eyles,D.W. (2004) Vitamin D3-implications for brain development. *J. Steroid Biochem. Mol. Biol.*, 89-90, 557-560.

[48] Nieves,J., Cosman,F., Herbert,J., Shen,V. and Lindsay,R. (1994) High prevalence of vitamin D deficiency and reduced bone mass in multiple sclerosis. *Neurology*, 44, 1687-1692.

[49] Munger,K.L., Levin,L.I., Hollis,B.W., Howard,N.S. and Ascherio,A. (2006) Serum 25-hydroxyvitamin D levels and risk of multiple sclerosis. *JAMA*, 296, 2832-2838.

[50] Munger,K.L., Zhang,S.M., O'Reilly,E., Hernan,M.A., Olek,M.J., Willett,W.C. et al. (2004) Vitamin D intake and incidence of multiple sclerosis. *Neurology*, 62, 60-65.

[51] Knekt,P., Kilkkinen,A., Rissanen,H., Marniemi,J., Saaksjarvi,K. and Heliovaara,M. (2010) Serum vitamin D and the risk of Parkinson disease. *Arch. Neurol.*, 67, 808-811.

[52] Hummer,M., Malik,P., Gasser,R.W., Hofer,A., Kemmler,G., Moncayo Naveda,R.C., et al. (2005) Osteoporosis in patients with schizophrenia. *Am. J. Psychiatry*, 162, 162-167.

[53] Kishimoto,T., Watanabe,K., Shimada,N., Makita,K., Yagi,G. and Kashima,H. (2008) Antipsychotic-induced hyperprolactinemia inhibits the hypothalamo-pituitary-gonadal axis and reduces bone mineral density in male patients with schizophrenia. *J. Clin. Psychiatry*, 69, 385-391.

[54] Schneider,B., Weber,B., Frensch,A., Stein,J. and Fritz,J. (2000) Vitamin D in schizophrenia, major depression and alcoholism. *J. Neural. Transm.*, 107, 839-842.

[55] Hummer,M., Malik,P., Gasser,R.W., Hofer,A., Kemmler,G., Moncayo Naveda,R.C., et al. (2005) Osteoporosis in patients with schizophrenia. *Am. J. Psychiatry*, 162, 162-167.

[56] Kishimoto,T., Watanabe,K., Shimada,N., Makita,K., Yagi,G. and Kashima,H. (2008) Antipsychotic-induced hyperprolactinemia inhibits the hypothalamo-pituitary-gonadal axis and reduces bone mineral density in male patients with schizophrenia. *J. Clin. Psychiatry*, 69, 385-391.

[57] McGrath,J.J., Eyles,D.W., Pedersen,C.B., Anderson,C., Ko,P., Burne,T.H., et al. (2010) Neonatal vitamin d status and risk of schizophrenia: a population-based case-control study. *Arch. Gen. Psychiatry*, 67, 889-894.

[58] McGrath,J. (1999) Hypothesis: is low prenatal vitamin D a risk-modifying factor for schizophrenia? *Schizophr. Res.*, 40, 173-177.

[59] Kay,S.R., Opler,L.A. and Lindenmayer,J.P. (1988) Reliability and validity of the positive and negative syndrome scale for schizophrenics. *Psychiatry Res.*, 23, 99-110.

[60] Hamilton,M. (1960) A rating scale for depression. *J Neurol. Neurosurg. Psychiatry*, 23, 56-62.

[61] Akahane,A. and Nanko,S. (2003) [Pathogenesis and heterogeneity in schizophrenia]. *Ryoikibetsu. Shokogun. Shirizu.*, 25-29.

[62] Sawa,A. and Snyder,S.H. (2002) Schizophrenia: diverse approaches to a complex disease. *Science*, 296, 692-695.

[63] Cherniack,E.P., Troen,B.R., Florez,H.J., Roos,B.A. and Levis,S. (2009) Some new food for thought: the role of vitamin D in the mental health of older adults. *Curr. Psychiatry Rep.*, 11, 12-19.

[64] Arnson,Y., Amital,H. and Shoenfeld,Y. (2007) Vitamin D and autoimmunity: new aetiological and therapeutic considerations. *Ann. Rheum. Dis.*, 66, 1137-1142.

[65] Holick,M.F. (2004) Sunlight and vitamin D for bone health and prevention of autoimmune diseases, cancers, and cardiovascular disease. *Am. J. Clin. Nutr.*, 80, 1678S-1688S.

[66] Holick,M.F. (2006) Vitamin D: its role in cancer prevention and treatment. *Prog. Biophys. Mol. Biol.*, 92, 49-59.

[67] Holick,M.F. (2007) Vitamin D deficiency. *N. Engl. J. Med.*, 357, 266-281.

[68] Hollis,B.W. (2008) Measuring 25-hydroxyvitamin D in a clinical environment: challenges and needs. *Am. J. Clin. Nutr.*, 88, 507S-510S.

[69] Souberbielle,J.C., Body,J.J., Lappe,J.M., Plebani,M., Shoenfeld,Y., Wang,T.J., et al. (2010) Vitamin D and musculoskeletal health, cardiovascular disease, autoimmunity and cancer: Recommendations for clinical practice. *Autoimmun. Rev.*, 9, 709-715.

[70] Pelajo, C.F., Lopez-Benitez,J.M. and Miller,L.C. (2010) Vitamin D and autoimmune rheumatologic disorders. *Autoimmun. Rev.*, 9, 507-510.

[71] Selmi, C. and Tsuneyama,K. (2010) Nutrition, geoepidemiology, and autoimmunity. *Autoimmun. Rev.*, 9, A267-A270.

[72] Milo,R. and Kahana,E. (2010) Multiple sclerosis: geoepidemiology, genetics and the environment. *Autoimmun. Rev.*, 9, A387-A394.

[73] Autier,P. and Gandini,S. (2007) Vitamin D supplementation and total mortality: a meta-analysis of randomized controlled trials. *Arch. Intern. Med.*, 167, 1730-1737.

[74] Giovannucci,E. (2007) Epidemiological evidence for vitamin D and colorectal cancer. *J. Bone Miner. Res.*, 22 Suppl 2, V81-V85.

[75] Giovannucci,E., Liu,Y., Hollis,B.W. and Rimm,E.B. (2008) 25-hydroxyvitamin D and risk of myocardial infarction in men: a prospective study. *Arch. Intern. Med.*, 168, 1174-1180.

[76] Giovannucci,E. (2008) Vitamin D status and cancer incidence and mortality. *Adv. Exp. Med. Biol.*, 624, 31-42.

[77] Arnson,Y., Amital,H. and Shoenfeld,Y. (2007) Vitamin D and autoimmunity: new aetiological and therapeutic considerations. *Ann. Rheum. Dis.*, 66, 1137-1142.

[78] Holick,M.F. (2007) Vitamin D deficiency. *N. Engl. J. Med.*, 357, 266-281.

[79] Carvalho,J.F., Blank,M., Kiss,E., Tarr,T., Amital,H. and Shoenfeld,Y. (2007) Anti-vitamin D, vitamin D in SLE: preliminary results. *Ann. N. Y. Acad. Sci.*, 1109, 550-557.

[80] Holick,M.F. (2007) Vitamin D deficiency. *N. Engl. J. Med.*, 357, 266-281.

[81] The Mosaic of Autoimmunity. Proceedings of a meeting in honor of Professor Shoenfeld in Tel Aviv, Israel, February 10-11, 2008. *Autoimmun. Rev.*, 7, 161-266.

[82] Cutolo,M. (2009) Vitamin D and autoimmune rheumatic diseases. *Rheumatology. (Oxford)*, 48, 210-212.

[83] Shoenfeld,N., Amital,H. and Shoenfeld,Y. (2009) The effect of melanism and vitamin D synthesis on the incidence of autoimmune disease. *Nat. Clin. Pract. Rheumatol.*, 5, 99-105.

[84] Vacca,A., Cormier,C., Piras,M., Mathieu,A., Kahan,A. and Allanore,Y. (2009) Vitamin D deficiency and insufficiency in 2 independent cohorts of patients with systemic sclerosis. *J. Rheumatol.*, 36, 1924-1929.

[85] Amital, H., Szekanecz,Z., Szucs,G., Danko,K., Nagy,E., Csepany,T. *et al.* (2010) Serum concentrations of 25-OH vitamin D in patients with systemic lupus erythematosus (SLE) are inversely related to disease activity: is it time to routinely supplement patients with SLE with vitamin D? *Ann. Rheum. Dis.*, 69, 1155-1157.

[86] Milo,R. and Kahana,E. (2010) Multiple sclerosis: geoepidemiology, genetics and the environment. *Autoimmun. Rev.*, 9, A387-A394.

[87] Shapira,Y., Agmon-Levin,N. and Shoenfeld,Y. (2010) Geoepidemiology of autoimmune rheumatic diseases. *Nat. Rev. Rheumatol.*, 6:468-76.

[88] Vieira,V.M., Hart,J.E., Webster,T.F., Weinberg,J., Puett,R., Laden,F., et al. (2010) Association between Residences in U.S. Northern Latitudes and Rheumatoid Arthritis: A Spatial Analysis of the Nurses' Health Study. *Environ. Health Perspect.*, 118, 957-961.

[89] Maverakis,E., Miyamura,Y., Bowen,M.P., Correa,G., Ono,Y. and Goodarzi,H. (2010) Light, including ultraviolet. *J. Autoimmun.*, 34, J247-J257.

[90] Motrich,R.D., van,E.E., Depovere,J., Riera,C.M., Rivero,V.E. and Mathieu,C. (2009) Impact of vitamin D receptor activity on experimental autoimmune prostatitis. *J. Autoimmun.*, 32, 140-148.

[91] van Halteren,A.G., Tysma,O.M., van,E.E., Mathieu,C. and Roep,B.O. (2004) 1alpha,25-dihydroxyvitamin D3 or analogue treated dendritic cells modulate human autoreactive T cells via the selective induction of apoptosis. *J. Autoimmun.*, 23, 233-239.

[92] Kay,S.R., Opler,L.A. and Lindenmayer,J.P. (1988) Reliability and validity of the positive and negative syndrome scale for schizophrenics. *Psychiatry Res.*, 23, 99-110.

[93] Aromaa,A., Raitasalo,R., Reunanen,A., Impivaara,O., Heliovaara,M., Knekt,P., et al. (1994) Depression and cardiovascular diseases. *Acta Psychiatr. Scand. Suppl*, 377, 77-82.

[94] Curkendall,S.M., Mo,J., Glasser,D.B., Rose,S.M. and Jones,J.K. (2004) Cardiovascular disease in patients with schizophrenia in Saskatchewan, Canada. *J. Clin. Psychiatry*, 65, 715-720.

[95] Amital, H. and Shoenfeld,Y. (1993) Autoimmunity and schizophrenia: an epiphenomenon or an etiology? *Isr. J. Med. Sci.*, 29, 593-597.

[96] Schwartz,M., Kormilachev,M., Kushnir,M., Weller,B., Rochas,M. and Toubi,E. (2009) Lupus anticoagulant and anticardiolipin antibodies in serum of patients treated with risperidone. *J. Clin. Psychiatry*, 70, 769-771.

[97] Sirota,P., Bogdanov,I., Katzav,A., Hershko,R. and Chapman,J. (2006) Reduced anticardiolipin antibodies in first episode and chronic schizophrenia. *Psychiatry Res.*, 144, 211-216.

In: Vitamin D Deficiency
Editors: V. Lerner and C. Miodownik
ISBN: 978-1-61470-964-0

Commentary

Vitamin D levels and Bisphosphonate Treatment in Patients with Paget's Disease of Bone

Stergios A. Polyzos*, Athanasios D. Anastasilakis, Polyzois Makras and Evangelos Terpos

Abstract

Hypocalcaemia and secondary hyperparathyroidism after treatment with bisphosphonates have been described in a variety of bone diseases, including osteoporosis, bone metastases and Paget's disease of bone (PDB). Hypocalcaemia seems to be more severe after treatment with the more potent, intravenous zoledronic acid, which is currently the treatment of choice for PDB. Bisphosphonates initially create a bone remodeling imbalance by strongly suppressing bone resorption, while bone formation remains unaffected. In this setting serum calcium may be decreased, but quickly restored, with the cost of a long-standing secondary hyperparathyroidism. The ability of the parathyroid gland to increase renal reabsorption of calcium and 1.25-dihydroxy vitamin D production and to stimulate osteoclasts prevents long term hypocalcaemia. However, the effect of parathyroid hormone (PTH) on osteoclasts is, at least partly, restricted in patients taking bisphosphonates. Secondary hyperparathyroidism is a potentially detrimental condition, especially in patients already suffering from another bone disease. Serum calcium and/or vitamin D deficiency should be restored before bisphosphonate treatment and calcium and vitamin D administration should be continued for longer after achieving normocalcemia, which may shorten the duration of secondary hyperparathyroidism.

* Corresponding author: Stergios Polyzos, MD, MSc, Second Medical Clinic, Medical School, Aristotle University of Thessaloniki, Ippokration Hospital, Thessaloniki, Greece.Address: 13 Simou Lianidi, 551 34 Thessaloniki, Greece Tel/Fax: +302310424710 E-mail: stergios@endo.gr.

Keywords: Bone turnover; hyperparathyroidism; hypocalcaemia; osteomalacia; Paget's disease; parathyroid hormone; zoledronic acid; vitamin D

Abbreviations

BP	bisphosphonate;
PAM	pamidronate;
PDB	Paget's disease of bone;
PTH	parathyroid hormone;
TSAP	total serum alkaline phosphatase;
ZOL	zoledronic acid

Introduction

Paget's disease of bone (PDB) is characterized by focally high bone remodeling, with abnormalities in all the phases of the remodeling cycle [1]. The primary abnormality is believed to lie in the regulation of osteoclasts, which are increased in both number and size. In response to the rapid bone resorption, bone formation is also accelerated; the bone formation rate can be as high as six- or seven-fold over normal [2].

However, the newly formed bone is chaotic, bone architecture and structure are disrupted and mechanical strength is decreased. The affected bones become larger and more sclerotic than normal, but of poor quality. As a consequence, various complications may occur, including bone pain, deformity, pathological fracture and secondary osteoarthritis [1,2].

The concept of relative vitamin D deficiency in patients with PDB was suggested long ago in an observational study of 14 patients with biopsy-proven PDB, where areas of bone with high turnover showed localized osteomalacia when the vitamin D levels were in the lower limits of the normal range [3]. However, the prevalence of vitamin D deficiency among patients with PDB remains largely unknown, depending on vitamin D cut-off and the study population.

PDB is more frequently diagnosed in the elderly [4], in whom vitamin D deficiency is also more common [5]. Although both diseases predispose to fractures, their combined action to fragility has not been studied yet.

The older bisphosphonates (BPs), mainly etidronate, strongly inhibit bone mineralization, thereby possibly triggering or aggravating osteomalacia [6]. Mineralization defects have also been described in patients with PDB treated with pamidronate (PAM) [7]. On the contrary, to our knowledge, there are no reported cases of osteomalacia induced by alendronate, risedronate or zoledronic acid (ZOL) in patients with PDB.

Bisphosphonates in Paget's Disease of Bone

The biochemical goal of treatment in PDB is the normalization of total serum alkaline phosphatase (TSAP) [8]. BPs are currently the drugs of choice for PDB [1,9]. BPs are internalized by osteoclasts and inhibit their action and affect their survival [1].

Compared to other BPs, the third-generation BP ZOL binds the hydroxyapatite with higher affinity, and manifests increased antiresorptive potency and prolonged effect on bone turnover [1,10], thereby currently being a first-line treatment for patients with PDB [1]. The therapeutic superiority of ZOL in PDB was established with a double-blind randomized controlled trial, which compared a single 5 mg infusion of ZOL with 60 days of treatment with risedronate 30 mg/day [11]. The superiority of ZOL in PDB was also shown versus PAM infusion [12]. It is highlighted that PAM or risedronate were established treatment for PDB before ZOL introduction in clinical practice.

Hypocalcaemia and Secondary Hyperparathyroidism after Bisphosphonate Treatment

Given that nitrogen-containing BPs are potent and prolonged inhibitors of osteoclastic bone resorption, hypocalcaemia and secondary hypoparathyroidism following their administration have been described in different bone diseases, including osteoporosis [13], PDB [11,14], juvenile Paget's disease [15], osteogenesis imperfecta [16], bone metastases [17] and bone loss following liver transplantation [18]. Risk factors for severe BP-induced hypocalcaemia are pre-existing hypoparathyroidism, vitamin D deficiency, hypomagnesemia, renal failure and gastrointestinal malabsorption [19,20]. Generally, the intravenous BPs, may cause symptomatic hypocalcaemia more often than orally administered BPs, usually within days after the infusion [21].

Specifically in PDB, asymptomatic hypocalcaemia with secondary hyperparathyroidism occurred in all patients with PDB (n=29) who received PAM infusion in a study [22]. Notably, the overall rise in parathyroid hormone (PTH) was accompanied by an increase in 1,25-dihydroxy vitamin D. It seems pathophysiologically rational, but it might result in vitamin D depletion, especially if vitamin D was not optimally restored. In another study, PAM infusion resulted in hypocalcaemia and secondary hyperparathyroidism, which were more striking in patients with higher disease activity [23]. Hypocalcaemia and secondary hyperparathyroidism have also been reported after orally administered risedronate in PDB [24]. Calcium decrease and PTH increase was greater with daily risedronate 30 mg compared to 20 mg or 10 mg [24]. In the above mentioned randomized controlled trial [11], 8 patients in ZOL group developed hypocalcaemia (asymptomatic in 6 of them) compared with only 1 case of symptomatic hypocalcaemia in the risedronate group. The decrease in mean serum calcium was observed at the 10th day and it was greater in the ZOL group. These changes resulted in serum PTH increase in both groups at three and six months, which was greater in the ZOL group [11]. Secondary hyperparathyroidism after a single ZOL infusion has also been observed in another study [14]. ZOL effectively managed PDB activity, but significant hypocalcaemia was observed in the third day. No patient experienced symptoms or signs of hypocalcaemia. Interestingly, PTH remained significantly increased by 90% (range 20%-252%) three months after ZOL infusion and returned to baseline levels at twelve months, although calcium was normalized by the tenth day in all patients [14]. This pattern of sustained PTH increase after BPs treatment, despite serum calcium normalization, has been also reported in other metabolic bone diseases including bone metastases [25].

There are two more case reports of severe, symptomatic hypocalcaemia following BPs treatment in patients with PDB [26,27] and one in juvenile Paget's disease [15]. A patient with PDB and post-surgical hypoparathyroidism developed symptomatic hypocalcaemia three days after PAM infusion, despite the administration of calcium and calcitriol supplements. Symptomatic hypocalcaemia was repeated after orally administered alendronate, 19 months after PAM [26]. The second patient developed symptomatic hypocalcaemia ten days after risedronate administration, despite calcium and vitamin D supplementation [27]. Similarly, a case of juvenile Paget's disease developed severe hypocalcaemia, hypophosphatemia and secondary hyperparathyroidism after ZOL infusion, despite co-treatment with calcium and alphacalcidol [15]. Notably, a mild hyperparathyroidism remained for at least 19 months after ZOL infusion, much longer than hypocalcaemia and hypophosphatemia. In the last two cases [15,27], serum 25-hydroxyvitamin D levels were within normal range, but not optimal, which could have deteriorated hypocalcaemia and elongated secondary hyperparathyroidism after BP treatment.

It seems that the increase in PTH after BP treatment is compensatory in order to maintain normocalcemia. The ability of the parathyroid gland to react prevents long term hypocalcaemia, by increasing renal reabsorption of calcium and 1,25-dihydroxyvitamin D production and by stimulating osteoclasts. The effect of PTH on the osteoclasts is partly restricted in patients taking BPs, depending on the potency of the BP [20]. Conversely, the increased PTH antagonizes the effect of BPs on bone in order to maintain serum calcium. Therefore, BP-induced hypocalcaemia often subsides, despite continuing BP therapy [21], with the cost of secondary hyperparathyroidism. The newer more potent nitrogen-containing BPs, such as ZOL, initially create a bone remodeling imbalance by strongly suppressing bone resorption while bone formation remains initially unaffected [27]. Secondary hyperparathyroidism is a potentially detrimental condition, especially in patients already suffering from other bone disease [20].

PDB is a disease of high bone turnover. Previous data showed that bone turnover is a significant determinant of the amount of BPs retained within bone in patients with PDB and those with higher disease activity retain more BPs, especially at skeletal locations with high turnover [28]. In line, greater efficacy of ZOL treatment was observed in patients with higher bone turnover compared to those with lower bone turnover [14]. Furthermore, patients with higher bone turnover experienced more striking hypocalcaemia and secondary hyperparathyroidism after PAM administration [23]. It has been hypothesized that vitamin D deficiency might affect pagetic bones more than non-pagetic ones, since the local high bone turnover in the former renders them more vulnerable to vitamin D deficiency than the latter [29].

To our knowledge, the effect of vitamin D and calcium supplementation on patients with PDB has not been studied yet, although there is indirect evidence from cases of coexistence of PDB and vitamin D deficiency due to gastrointestinal malabsorption (steatorrhea) [29] or malnutrition [30]. Vitamin D deficiency can result in an elevation of TSAP, thus masking the diagnosis and implicating monitoring of PDB [31]. Vitamin D deficiency can result in poor mineralization of the newly-formed osteoid in affected bone, further weakening an already weak bone. Radionuclide bone scan cannot distinguish between Looser's zone and PDB-induced microfractures, thereby making it difficult to assess the actual extent of PDB [31].

Recommendations and Perspectives

Serum 25-hydroxy-vitamin D should be measured before BP administration, given that normal serum calcium, phosphate and PTH cannot exclude vitamin D deficiency. Pre-existing hypocalcaemia and vitamin D deficiency should be corrected before treatment with BPs, especially in PDB, where high bone turnover may easier result in severe hypocalcaemia. It is suggested that vitamin D should be optimally restored (> 25-30 ng/mL [32]), before BP administration. Even in normocalcemic patients without vitamin D deficiency, daily supplementation with calcium carbonate (500–1000 mg) and vitamin D (400–800 IU) before BP administration is recommended, in order to prevent hypocalcaemia and secondary hyperparathyroidism [1,9,20]. Vitamin D administration may attenuate PTH peak, thereby minimizing PTH action on the osteoclast function [33].

Despite these measures, hypocalcaemia may still develop after BP treatment in PDB [11,14,15,27]. In case of severe hypocalcaemia, standard protocol of intravenous calcium administration together with high doses of alphacalcidol or calcitriol may be needed [34]. Even if not severe, BP-induced secondary hyperparathyroidism may persist for long after restoring normocalcemia [14,15,27]. Thus, it is suggested that calcium and vitamin D administration, if not contraindicated, should be continued for longer after achieving normocalcemia, as in the management of osteoporosis, which may shorten the duration of secondary hyperparathyroidism [20]. However, these recommendations are based on indirect evidence, because there are no clinical trials investigating the effect of vitamin D supplements on BP-induced hypocalcaemia and secondary hyperparathyroidism.

Conclusion

BPs are currently the cornerstone in the management of PDB. However, BP-induced hypocalcaemia and secondary hyperparathyroidism should always be considered. Serum calcium, magnesium, PTH and vitamin D should be measured and optimally restored before BP treatment. Vitamin D-focused clinical trials would be of paramount importance in PDB, because if our speculations were validated, vitamin D would be rendered an inexpensive ally in BP-induced hypocalcaemia and secondary hyperparathyroidism, thereby resulting in more effective treatment of PDB.

References

[1] Polyzos,SA; Anastasilakis,AD; Terpos,E. Paget's disease of bone: emphasis on treatment with zoledronic acid. *Expert Rev. Endocrinol. Metabolism,* 2009 4; 424-434.

[2] Cundy,T; Bolland,M. Paget disease of bone. *Trends Endocrinol Metab,* 2008 19; 246-253.

[3] Williams,ED; Barr,WT; Rajan,KT. Relative vitamin D deficiency in Paget's disease. *Lancet,* 1981 1; 384-385.

[4] Cooper,C; Harvey,NC; Dennison,EM; van Staa,TP. Update on the epidemiology of Paget's disease of bone. *J. Bone Miner Res.,* 2006 21 Suppl 2; 3-8.

[5] Lanham-New,SA; Buttriss,JL; Miles,LM, et al. Proceedings of the Rank Forum on Vitamin D. *Br. J. Nutr.,* 2011 105; 144-156.

[6] Sparidans,RW; Twiss,IM; Talbot,S. Bisphosphonates in bone diseases. *Pharm World Sci,* 1998 20; 206-213.

[7] Adamson,BB; Gallacher,SJ; Byars,J; Ralston,SH; Boyle,IT; Boyce,BF. Mineralisation defects with pamidronate therapy for Paget's disease. *Lancet,* 1993 342; 1459-1460.

[8] Shankar,S; Hosking,DJ. Biochemical assessment of Paget's disease of bone. *J. Bone Miner Res.,* 2006 21 Suppl 2; 22-27.

[9] Devogelaer,JP; Bergmann,P; Body,JJ, et al. Management of patients with Paget's disease: a consensus document of the Belgian Bone Club. *Osteoporos Int.,* 2008 19; 1109-1117.

[10] Nancollas,GH; Tang,R; Phipps,RJ, et al. Novel insights into actions of bisphosphonates on bone: differences in interactions with hydroxyapatite. *Bone,* 2006 38; 617-627.

[11] Reid,IR; Miller,P; Lyles,K, et al. Comparison of a single infusion of zoledronic acid with risedronate for Paget's disease. *N. Engl. J. Med.,* 2005 353; 898-908.

[12] Hosking,D; Lyles,K; Brown,JP, et al. Long-term control of bone turnover in Paget's disease with zoledronic acid and risedronate. *J. Bone Miner Res.,* 2007 22; 142-148.

[13] Harris,ST; Gertz,BJ; Genant,HK, et al. The effect of short term treatment with alendronate on vertebral density and biochemical markers of bone remodeling in early postmenopausal women. *J. Clin. Endocrinol. Metab.,* 1993 76; 1399-1406.

[14] Avramidis,A; Polyzos,SA; Moralidis,E, et al. Scintigraphic, biochemical, and clinical response to zoledronic acid treatment in patients with Paget's disease of bone. *J. Bone Miner Metab.,* 2008 26; 635-641.

[15] Polyzos,SA; Anastasilakis,AD; Litsas,I, et al. Profound hypocalcaemia following effective response to zoledronic acid treatment in a patient with juvenile Paget's disease. *J. Bone Miner Metab.,* 2010 28; 706-712.

[16] Vuorimies,I; Toiviainen-Salo,S; Hero,M; Makitie,O. Zoledronic Acid Treatment in Children with Osteogenesis Imperfecta. *Horm. Res. Paediatr.,* 2011 (epub ahead of print).

[17] Sayin,M; Yazici,G. Hyperparathyroidism secondary to zoledronic acid infusion: case report. *Support Care Cancer,* 2009 17; 469-470.

[18] Crawford, BA; Kam,C; Pavlovic,J, et al. Zoledronic acid prevents bone loss after liver transplantation: a randomized, double-blind, placebo-controlled trial. *Ann. Intern. Med.,* 2006 144; 239-248.

[19] Chennuru,S; Koduri,J; Baumann,MA. Risk factors for symptomatic hypocalcaemia complicating treatment with zoledronic acid. *Intern Med. J.,* 2008 38; 635-637.

[20] Polyzos,SA; Anastasilakis,AD; Terpos,E. Transient secondary hyperparathyroidism following intravenous infusion of zoledronic acid. *Support Care Cancer,* 2009 17; 1329-1330.

[21] Papapetrou,PD. Bisphosphonate-associated adverse events. *Hormones (Athens),* 2009 8; 96-110.

[22] Fenton,AJ; Gutteridge,DH; Kent,GN, et al. Intravenous aminobisphosphonate in Paget's disease: clinical, biochemical, histomorphometric and radiological responses. *Clin. Endocrinol. (Oxf),* 1991 34; 197-204.

[23] Gutteridge,DH; Retallack,RW; Ward,LC, et al. Clinical, biochemical, hematologic, and radiographic responses in Paget's disease following intravenous pamidronate disodium: a 2-year study. *Bone,* 1996 19; 387-394.

[24] Brown,JP; Hosking,DJ; Ste-Marie,L, et al. Risedronate, a highly effective, short-term oral treatment for Paget's disease: a dose-response study. *Calcif. Tissue Int.,* 1999 64; 93-99.

[25] Sayin,M; Yazici,G. Hyperparathyroidism secondary to zoledronic acid infusion: case report. *Support Care Cancer,* 2009 17; 469-470.

[26] Stuckey,BG; Lim,EM; Kent,GN; Ward,LC; Gutteridge,DH. Bisphosphonate therapy for Paget's disease in a patient with hypoparathyroidism: profound hypocalcaemia, rapid response, and prolonged remission. *J. Bone Miner Res.,* 2001 16; 1719-1723.

[27] Whitson,HE; Lobaugh,B; Lyles,KW. Severe hypocalcaemia following bisphosphonate treatment in a patient with Paget's disease of bone. *Bone,* 2006 39; 954-958.

[28] Cremers,SC; Eekhoff,ME; Den,HJ; Hamdy,NA; Vermeij,P; Papapoulos,SE. Relationships between pharmacokinetics and rate of bone turnover after intravenous bisphosphonate (olpadronate) in patients with Paget's disease of bone. *J. Bone Miner Res.,* 2003 18; 868-875.

[29] Nagant de Deuxchaisnes,C; Maldague,B; Malghem,J; Devogelaer,JP; Huaux,JP; Romboutslindemans,C. The Action of the Main Therapeutic Regimes on Pagets-Disease of Bone, with A Note on the Effect of Vitamin-D Deficiency. *Arthritis and Rheumatism,* 1980 23; 1215-1232.

[30] de Seze,S; Durand,C. Maladie de Paget et Carence Calcique. *Rev Rhum,* 1945 12; 193-217.

[31] Kannan,S; Mahadevan,S; Sathya,A; Sriram,U. A tale of three diseases of the bone. *Singapore Med. J.,* 2008 49; 263-265.

[32] Heaney,RP; Dowell,MS; Hale,CA; Bendich,A. Calcium absorption varies within the reference range for serum 25-hydroxyvitamin D. *J. Am. Coll Nutr.,* 2003 22; 142-146.

[33] Stewart,GO; Gutteridge,DH; Price,RI, et al. Prevention of appendicular bone loss in Paget's disease following treatment with intravenous pamidronate disodium. *Bone,* 1999 24; 139-144.

[34] Cooper,MS; Gittoes,NJ. Diagnosis and management of hypocalcaemia. *BMJ,* 2008 336; 1298-1302.

Index

A

F

G

H

I

K

L

N

O

P

Q

R

S

T